Portfolio Guidance for Ve

T0249660

THE COLLEGE OF
ANIMAL WELFARE

For Butterworth-Heinemann:

Senior Commissioning Editor: Mary Seager
Development Editor: Catharine Steers
Project Manager: Gail Wright
Designer: Andy Chapman
Project Management and Typesetting: Temple Design

Portfolio Guidance for Veterinary Nurses

The College of Animal Welfare

SECOND EDITION

Butterworth-Heinemann

BUTTERWORTH-HEINEMANN
An imprint of Elsevier Science Limited

First edition 2000
Second edition 2003

ISBN 0 7506 5640 9

British Library Cataloguing in Publication Data
A catalogue record for this book is available from the British Library

Library of Congress Cataloging in Publication Data
A catalog record for this book is available from the Library of Congress

Note
Veterinary knowledge is constantly changing. As new information becomes available, changes in treatment, procedures, equipment and the use of drugs become necessary. The author and the publishers have taken care to ensure that the information given in this text is accurate and up to date. However, readers are strongly advised to confirm that the information, especially with regard to drug usage, complies with the latest legislation and standards of practice.

ELSEVIER SCIENCE
your source for books,
journals and multimedia
in the health sciences
www.elsevierhealth.com

The publisher's policy is to use paper manufactured from sustainable forests

Printed and bound by Antony Rowe Ltd, Eastbourne
Transferred to digital printing 2005

Contents

Introduction

The Royal College of Veterinary Surgeons (RCVS) Veterinary Nurse Training Scheme changed in January 1999 to become focused around Scottish/National Vocational Qualifications (S/NVQs). This change permitted the development of national standards for veterinary nursing, improving the skills of the workforce and promoting an improved standard of nursing care and practice.

Since this change, each student nurse has been required to complete a portfolio of evidence that demonstrates his or her standards of nursing within practice. It is used to provide evidence that the student has achieved the occupational standard for the S/NVQ in Veterinary Nursing, in addition to providing a useful record of performance for future employment.

The first edition of the Veterinary Nursing Portfolio was published in 1998 and revised in 2001. The third edition has just been approved by the RCVS. *Portfolio Guidance for Veterinary Nurses* second edition reflects the most up-to-date curriculum.

The aim of this book is to support the documentation produced by the RCVS and thereby assist both student veterinary nurses and their assessors in the completion of edition two of the portfolio. It will also be of use to those starting on edition three when it becomes available as, although not identical, the underlying principles of portfolio completion will remain the same.

1 History of veterinary nurse training and assessment

Since 1961, when the first training and assessment programme for veterinary nurses was launched on a national basis, over 6400 students have qualified as veterinary nurses. Originally known as Registered Animal Nursing Auxiliary (RANA), the title was changed in 1984 to that of Veterinary Nurse when a change in legislation removed the protection of the title 'Nurse', originally permitted to be used only by members of the General Nursing Council.

Occupational standards for veterinary nursing have been developed and piloted by the Veterinary Lead Body since 1993, the aim being to develop standards that reflect the roles and responsibilities of the veterinary nurse, and to outline those required for competent performance. Development of the standards was achieved through consultation with representatives of the veterinary and veterinary nursing professions.

Methods of assessment were then developed with the aim of maintaining the rigour of the existing professional examination whilst including practice-based assessment of performance and knowledge. This led to the development of the objective syllabus and practice portfolio.

2 The new veterinary nurse scheme

The new scheme is based upon practice training and assessment combined with an independent examination-based assessment (i.e. the RCVS VN examination). It normally takes two years to qualify as a veterinary nurse and this now leads to the S/NVQ at Levels 2 and 3 when completed.

2.1 Enrolment

The following are the current requirements laid down by the RCVS for enrolment on the Veterinary Nurse Scheme:

- Be a minimum of 17 years of age.
- Hold a minimum of 5 GCSEs at grade C or above (or equivalent, e.g. the Pre-Veterinary Nursing Certificate). These must include English Language and either two science subjects or a science subject and mathematics.
- Be employed at a practice that is a veterinary nurse Training and Assessment Centre (VNAC) or a Training Practice (TP), or be a student on a Veterinary Nursing degree course. (See Appendix A for an explanation of the changes that are currently affecting the approval of practices for veterinary nurse training.)

2.2 Training

The student veterinary nurse (SVN) must be employed at a VNAC or TP for a minimum of 94 weeks (full-time employment), including annual leave and sickness absence. Full-time employment should be considered as no less than 35 contracted hours per week (not including on-call hours and overtime). Part-time employment should equate to a minimum period of 165 weeks, including annual leave and sickness absence. Part-time employment should be considered as no less than 20 contracted hours per week (not including on-call hours and overtime).

SVNs may choose to support their training in practice with educational courses, which may be full-time block release courses, part-time day release courses or distance learning programmes. The RCVS emphasise that, although it is not a mandatory requirement of veterinary nurse training, educational programmes that provide the underpinning knowledge of the S/NVQ are recommended. They assist the student with the theory relating to practice, which in turn should improve the quality of nursing care, assisting the student to achieve competence for the S/NVQ assessment.

2.3 Assessment

2.3.1 Practice-based assessment
Each student veterinary nurse is assessed on different activities within the VNAC/TP. These activities are those detailed in the occupational standards and are recorded in the portfolio as evidence that the national standard has been met.

2.3.2 Independent assessment
This consists of:

● A written examination (consisting of two papers of multiple choice questions), which takes place during Part 1 training (towards the S/NVQ Level 2) and at the end of Part 2 training (towards S/NVQ Level 3).

- A practical examination of key practical skills which is taken at the end of Part 2 training (towards S/NVQ Level 3).
- External verification of the practice portfolio, which occurs in two stages. The first external verification takes place after completion of portfolio modules 1–5 (in edition 1; modules 1– 4 in edition 2; modules 1–5 in edition 3), i.e. NVQ Level 2 (Part 1). The second external verification takes place after completion of modules 6–14 (in edition 1; modules 5–10 in edition 2; modules 6–11 in edition 3), i.e. NVQ Level 3 (Part 2).

Depending upon the training status of the practice (i.e. whether an ATAC or a TP), the requirements for external verification will differ. Students at ATACs will need to submit their portfolios to the RCVS for external verification. Students at TPs will be requested to submit their portfolios for internal verification by their VNAC, following which a sample will be seen by the external verifier. The RCVS administer all aspects of the independent assessment.

2.4 Qualification

The student achieves the S/NVQ Level 2 on successful completion of portfolio modules 1–5 (in edition 1; modules 1–4 in edition 2; modules 1–5 in edition 3) and the Part 1 examination. They complete S/NVQ Level 3 on successful completion of portfolio modules 6–14 (in edition 1; modules 5–10 in edition 2; modules 6–11 in edition 3) and the Part 2 written and practical examinations. Only following successful completion of S/NVQ Levels 2 and 3, and stipulated practice hours, does a student qualify as a veterinary nurse and become eligible to enter their name on the RCVS list of veterinary nurses.

3 Scottish/National Vocational Qualifications (S/NVQs)

3.1 History of S/NVQs

In order to fully appreciate and work with the veterinary nursing S/NVQs, it is necessary to become familiar with the structure and function of S/NVQs as a whole.

S/NVQs are qualifications based upon occupational standards developed by industry representatives. The standards for the veterinary nursing S/NVQs were developed by the Veterinary Lead Body, which includes veterinary, veterinary nursing and allied industry representatives.

The Veterinary Lead Body conducted a detailed analysis of the sector and the job roles therein. From this analysis they were able to determine the main roles and responsibilities of the veterinary nurse, and develop standards reflecting these roles. These standards show the outcome of competent performance, including the knowledge and understanding required to achieve the outcome.

The standards are composed of a number of different units, representing the key roles of the veterinary nurse. Each unit is further broken down into *elements* which are each composed of *performance criteria* (what the veterinary nurse should be able to do) and *knowledge and understanding* (what the veterinary nurse needs to know and understand relating to the element). This can best be represented by Figure 3.1.

S/NVQs can exist at Levels 1–5, although in the context of veterinary nursing at the time of writing, they are available at Levels 2 and 3. The level of the S/NVQ is defined by the responsibilities of the job role as detailed overleaf:

Level 1 Work requires the person to perform a range of routine activities under supervision.

Level 2 The person is required to perform a range of routine and non-routine activities within their work, with limited supervision.

Level 3 The job role requires performance of a wide range of skilled and complex tasks and also includes responsibility for the supervision of others.

Level 4 Operating at managerial level, with the responsibility for controlling staff and resources.

Level 5 Operating at a senior professional level and being responsible for planning, policy development and the strategic management of the organisation.

To qualify as a veterinary nurse, eligible for entry on the RCVS veterinary nurse list, students (or candidates – the terminology used for an individual working towards an S/NVQ) must complete Levels 2 and 3 of the veterinary nursing S/NVQ and stipulated practice hours.

Fig 3.1: Structure of the veterinary nursing S/NVQs

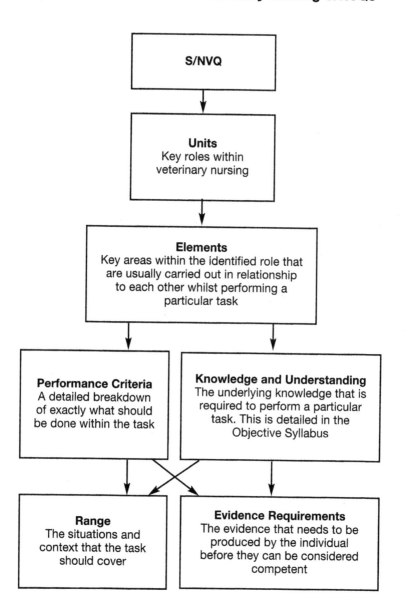

4 Accrediting and awarding bodies

Once occupational standards have been finalised by the Occupational Lead Body (e.g. the Veterinary Lead Body), they are submitted to the accrediting body for approval as S/NVQs. The accrediting bodies are:

● The Qualifications Curriculum Authority (QCA) for NVQs in England, Wales and Northern Ireland.
● The Scottish Qualifications Authority (SQA) for SVQs in Scotland.

These should not be confused with the awarding body, which, in the case of veterinary nursing, is the RCVS. As an awarding body, the RCVS is responsible for:

● The development and review of assessment systems.
● Maintenance of quality assurance of the qualification, administration and certification procedures.
● Marketing and promotional activities.

They are also responsible for the approval of centres to offer the S/NVQs (changes to the approval of centres for the training of SVNs are detailed in Appendix A). These centres are known as Veterinary Nurse Assessment Centres (VNACs) and are required by the RCVS to have access to a range of resources within their own TPs, a sample of which can be found in the RCVS Training Centre Handbook.

5 Key roles and responsibilities in the delivery of S/NVQs

5.1 The people involved

Candidate: The candidate the individual undertaking the S/NVQ. They have to be able to demonstrate that they are competent with regard to the occupational standards. In the context of veterinary nursing, the candidate is the student veterinary nurse who is working towards their S/NVQ Levels 2 and 3 in veterinary nursing.

Assessor: The assessor is the person who assesses the candidate against occupational standards to determine competency. Occasionally there may be more than one assessor per candidate. The assessor should monitor the candidate's progress throughout the S/NVQ by planning assessment strategies and identifying assessment opportunities within the workplace. They should also help identify appropriate training for the candidate to assist them in achieving the occupational standards.

Internal verifier: The internal verifier (or IV) is the person responsible for checking that the assessor(s) are assessing consistently and fairly (between different candidates and assessors) against the occupational standards. They may be from within the same practice as the assessor(s), or from a VNAC providing internal verification duties and support to a number of practices and assessors.

External verifier: The external verifier (or EV) is employed by the awarding body, in this case the RCVS. They are responsible for verifying the assessment and verification decisions made by the assessor and internal verifier at centres around the country, thereby ensuring that the standard is consistent between centres.

5.2 Assessment

In order to deliver the S/NVQs, all VNACs/TPs must have access to appropriately qualified and trained assessors, to assess the student veterinary nurse (SVN) against the occupational standards to determine competence.

The QCA/SQA and the RCVS determine requirements for assessors. To be an assessor for the veterinary nursing S/NVQs the individual must:

- be a qualified veterinary nurse, whose name is maintained on the list held by the RCVS; or
- be a veterinary surgeon (MRCVS).

Each assessor should also hold, or be working towards, Units D32 and/or D33 from the training and development S/NVQ of the Training and Development Lead Body (TDLB, now part of the Employment National Training Organisation).

These units are an important part of the S/NVQ assessment procedure. They provide evidence that the assessor is trained to assess candidates' performance (Unit D32) and/or assess candidates using differing sources of evidence (Unit D33) in a fair and consistent manner. They are a requirement of all assessors who assess S/NVQs, no matter what the occupational role.

The RCVS currently recommend that assessors should have held their professional qualification for a minimum of 12 months prior to taking on the role of assessor.

Trainee assessors should have all their assessment decisions countersigned by a qualified assessor or internal verifier.

5.2.1 Responsibilities of the assessor

The assessor is responsible for planning and conducting assessments with the SVN (or candidate) and maintaining accurate records of all such assessments. They should provide feedback to the SVN regarding their assessments and help to implement an appropriate corrective action plan should the standard not have been achieved on assessment. They should regularly review and monitor the progress of the SVN, discussing and agreeing any changes to the student's individual assessment plan that may be necessary. They should assist the SVN with the collection and presentation of evidence in the portfolio to support the assessment procedures.

5.3 Verification

There are two forms of verification, internal and external.

5.3.1 Internal verification

The internal verifier (or IV) may exist within the practice or VNAC itself. In some circumstances the IV may be external to the practice (a TP) and will be allocated to the TP by the VNAC, to come in when necessary to carry out the internal verification procedures required by the RCVS.

The QCA/SQA and the RCVS determine requirements for IVs. To be an IV for the veterinary nursing S/NVQs the individual must:

- be a qualified veterinary nurse, listed in the RCVS veterinary nurse register; or
- be a veterinary surgeon (MRCVS).

Each IV should also hold, or be working towards, Unit D34 (and preferably Units D32 and/or D33) from the training and development S/NVQ of the Training and Development Lead

Body (TDLB, now part of the Employment National Training Organisation).

Unit D34 is an important part of the S/NVQ verification procedure. It provides evidence that the IV is trained to internally verify the assessment process in a fair and consistent manner. It is a requirement of all IVs who verify S/NVQs, no matter what the occupational role.

5.3.2 Responsibilities of the internal verifier

The IV is responsible for the verification (checking) of the assessment practice of assessors. They should sample evidence from all assessors, ensuring that they cover all different forms of assessment used to verify the competence of candidates. During this process they should maintain accurate records of their internal verification. They are also responsible for liaising with assessors, identifying any training needs and co-ordinating the activity of the assessors within the VNAC/TP through regular update meetings. They are also the first point of contact with the external verifier for the VNAC/TP.

5.3.3 External verification

The external verifier (or EV) is employed by the RCVS to carry out external verification procedures across a number of VNACs on a national basis. The QCA/SQA and the RCVS determine requirements for EVs. To be an EV for the veterinary nursing S/NVQs the individual must:

- be a qualified, listed veterinary nurse; or,
- be a veterinary surgeon (MRCVS).

Each EV should also hold, or be working towards, Unit D35 from the training and development S/NVQ of the Training and Development Lead Body (TDLB, now part of the

Employment National Training Organisation).

This unit is an important part of the S/NVQ verification procedure. It provides evidence that the EV is trained to externally verify the assessment process in a fair and consistent manner. It is a requirement of all EVs who verify S/NVQs, no matter what the occupational role.

External verification by the RCVS ensures that all veterinary nursing portfolios meet a minimum standard regarding the evidence contained. The EV examines case log sheets and other evidence to ensure that sufficient evidence has been supplied to support the assessor's decision that the SVN has met the national standard.

5.3.4 Responsibilities of the external verifier

The EV is responsible for monitoring the activities of VNACs on a national basis. They sample assessment practice and evidence to ensure that the standards are being met. This may involve direct observation of assessments, review of portfolios as well as discussions with SVNs, assessors and the IV. On completion of the appropriate modules of the veterinary nurse portfolio, the EV verifies the modules before the S/NVQ certificate can be issued. They are responsible for sampling the VNACs' internal verification methods as a means of quality control for the qualification.

EVs are responsible for supporting the VNAC during the initial implementation of the S/NVQs and subsequently advising as and when the need arises. They may choose to hold workshops for IVs and assessors to assist with this process and to provide networking opportunities for VNACs.

6 Changes to D units

The occupational standards and units from the training and development suite of qualifications are, at the time of writing, under review. They have been accredited as A and V units. It is likely that any assessor or verifier with the D units will not have to complete the A or V units, but will have to demonstrate professional updating in the context of the new units.

7 The veterinary nurse portfolio

The portfolio was introduced by the RCVS to assist both the SVN (candidate) and the assessor in the collection of evidence towards the veterinary nursing S/NVQs and should be used in conjunction with the occupational standards in the Training Centre Handbook.

It should be borne in mind that the nature of the portfolio and the diversity of veterinary practices will naturally produce different styles of portfolio. This is taken into consideration during the internal and external verification processes.

7.1 Portfolio structure and content
(2nd edition, 2001)

The portfolio (second edition) is divided into a number of sections. Section A explains work-based assessment, section B covers independent assessment and section C explains certification. Annexes include supporting documentation for the portfolio and guidance notes for case log completion. The portfolio should also be accompanied by a set of the occupational standards and the objective syllabus.

A portfolio coversheet should be completed with the relevant details, including name, enrolment number, date of enrolment, home address and postcode. This forms the front page of the portfolio that is submitted to the RCVS for external verification, or to the VNAC for internal verification.

Each page of the submitted portfolio should be numbered and recorded on a contents sheet (annex B). This provides an easy point of reference and is useful for cross-referencing.

A record of VN training for the candidate should be completed and submitted as part of the portfolio (annex C). This should include details of employment history, including any changes in employment, and details of college-based training undertaken. The RCVS may request submission of the record of training at any point during the candidate's time as a SVN – consequently it should be kept up to date at all times.

A signature authentication sheet should be completed by all those signatories in the portfolio. This includes the internal verifier, assessors, evidence gatherers (if appropriate) and the principal of the practice (annex D). It is advisable to complete this sheet as the SVN progresses through the portfolio. Should a member of the practice who has been involved with the portfolio leave without signing this sheet, it could take some time to track them down for an authentication signature.

Tracking sheets should be reviewed and updated regularly (annex E) along with the assessment planning and tutorial records (annex F). This provides an opportunity for the assessor and SVN to plan evidence gathering and assessment. This is a working document and it should be reviewed regularly. Obviously there may be situations where planned evidence gathering and assessments may be delayed, perhaps due to a particularly busy period within the surgery. This should be indicated on the plan and rescheduled for a later date.

The RCVS and VNAC must be informed if the SVN moves to a new practice. The form provided in annex C should be used.

Case log sheets for completion and assessment ensure that the VN occupational standards are met (annex G). The case log sheets for the different modules of the portfolio should be photocopied before use. Alternatively, the portfolio is available on the Internet at the RCVS website (www.rcvs.org.uk) for those students who wish to word process their evidence. Take care that the correct second edition of the portfolio is downloaded, as both are available.

The Level 2 modules include:
- Reception and client support
- Preparing for and assisting with non-surgical procedures
- Basic nursing
- Health, safety and security.

The Level 3 modules include:
- Laboratory and diagnostic aids
- Medical nursing and fluid therapy
- Radiography
- Surgical nursing and theatre practice
- Anaesthesia
- Maintenance of the availability of veterinary resources.

Each module has four parts:
- Guidance notes
- Evidence requirements
- Case log sheets
- Module assessment summary sheet.

Take care to read parts 1 and 2, and complete enough of each case log to fulfil the evidence requirements.

The RCVS are, at the time of writing, developing a third edition of the portfolio. This is currently in draft form and may be subject to some minor alterations; however, the overall structure and module titles remain the same. There has been some alteration to reflect the changes to VNACs and TPs in the portfolio guidance notes, and the case log sheets are presented in landscape rather than portrait format. It is important to note that whichever edition of the portfolio is used, care should be taken not to mix the log sheets and guidance notes between different editions. However, it is possible to change editions between NVQ Level 2 and NVQ Level 3 if desired.

Edition 3 of the portfolio includes:

MODULE 1
Health and safety and personal performance	*Total = 3 case logs*
1a Health and safety risk assessment	*1 case log*
1b Health and safety for self and others	*1 case log*
1c Establish and maintain working relationships with others	*1 case log*

MODULE 2
Reception and client support	*Total = 7 case logs*
2a Reception duties	*1 case log*
2b Dispensing medication to animals	*4 case logs*
2c Providing detailed information to clients	*2 case logs*

MODULE 3
Admit and discharge animals	*Total = 4 case logs*
3a Admit animals for veterinary procedures	*2 case logs*
3b Discharge animals after veterinary treatment	*2 case logs*

MODULE 4
Prepare for and assist with veterinary non-surgical procedures and investigations	*Total = 5 case logs*
4a Prepare for and assist with medical procedures and investigations	*5 case logs*

MODULE 5
Basic nursing	*Total = 15 case logs*
5a Basic animal management	*7 case logs*
5b Basic first aid	*3 case logs*
5c Administration of medication	*5 case logs*

S/NVQ Level 2 requires completion of modules 1–5 with a total of 34 case log sheets.

MODULE 6
Laboratory and diagnostic aids	*Total = 7 case logs*
6a Laboratory and diagnostic aids	*5 case logs*
6b Maintenance of equipment	*1 case log*
6c Health and safety assessment	*1 case log*

MODULE 7
Medical nursing and fluid therapy	*Total = 9 case logs + 2 expanded reports*
7a Medical nursing	*6 case logs + 2 expanded reports*
7b Fluid therapy	*3 case logs*

MODULE 8
Diagnostic imaging	*Total = 10 case logs*
8a Radiography	*8 case logs*
8b Health and safety risk assessment	*1 case log*
8c Ultrasound or endoscopy	*1 case log*

MODULE 9
Surgical nursing and theatre practice	*Total = 12 case logs + 2 expanded reports*
9a Maintain asepsis	*1 case log*
9b Sterilisation	*2 case logs*
9c Surgical nursing	*6 case logs + 2 expanded reports*
9d Maintenance of equipment	*3 case logs*

MODULE 10
Anaesthesia	*Total = 8 case logs*
10a Anaesthesia record	*6 case logs*
10b Health and safety risk assessment – anaesthesia	*1 case log*
10c Anaesthetic emergency box	*1 case log*

MODULE 11
Manage the availability of veterinary resources	*Total = 2 case logs*
11a Maintain the supply of veterinary materials	*1 case log*
11b Maintain the availability of veterinary equipment	*1 case log*

S/NVQ Level 3 requires the completion of modules 6–11 with a total of 48 case logs and 4 expanded reports.

8 General guidelines for the veterinary nurse portfolio

8.1 Case logs should be written up as soon as possible in order that the assessor can give feedback and complete their comments. All sheets should be presented either neatly hand-written in blue or black ballpoint pen (since pencil does not constitute a permanent record), or word processed.

8.2 Any client details (name and address) should be removed to protect client confidentiality (therefore these should not be used for case number identification). Case number identification should be the practice reference, however where this is the client details then a suitable alternative should be used. A copy of the chosen method of log referencing relating to client details should be maintained (which should not be submitted with the portfolio). This will allow the candidate to relate back to original practice records if required e.g. for completion of the Level 3 modules of the portfolio.

8.3 Evidence from the treatment of large animals (equines and farm animal species) should not be used within the portfolio, unless the SVN is working towards the equine route.

8.4 Where necessary, to avoid the duplication of information, appendices may be used and cross-referenced between case logs (but only where relevant).

E.g. When considering the use of appendices in the Basic Animal Management (BAM) case logs in the Basic Nursing module:

Appendix BAM 1.1   Cleaning Protocol

could be used in the first BAM case log and referred to in subsequent logs where appropriate,

Appendix BAM 1.2   Bedding Protocol

as above.

8.5 Each log sheet should have the name of the SVN, the SVN's signature and enrolment number, and be signed and dated by the assessor when competency has been achieved. Comments from both the SVN and assessor must also be included to reflect the SVN's own role in the case, and evidence of assessment to the occupational standard by the assessor.

8.6 Evidence can be recorded in sentence form or as bullet points, as long as major points are clarified. Consideration should be given to the space provided and clarity of presentation. Large quantities of 'waffle'/irrelevant information are not considered appropriate. Where necessary, an additional sheet, firmly attached and neatly and clearly laid out with the appropriate heading and numbering, should be used. If additional sheets are attached, these should be recorded at the foot of the case log sheet to prevent them being overlooked or misplaced.

8.7 Where a reference to a particular drug is made within the evidence of any unit (case log or written report) the generic name should be used.

8.8 'Student comments' must include the role that was played by the student in the case, e.g. sole charge for nursing care, and any other relevant information that the student may wish to contribute, such as the student's general observations. 'Student comments' should be judged by the assessor. This section must be completed.

8.9 The assessor's statement should indicate how the assessor came to the conclusion that the student was competent, i.e. a brief meaningful comment on the student's performance. This will need reference to the occupational standards in the handbook. This section must be completed. The assessor may state that they questioned the candidate on an aspect of the log sheet and these questions were answered correctly. This indicates evidence of knowledge and understanding and is also evidence of ongoing assessment. The question record may be included.

9 Guidance notes for modules 1–4 (Edition 2)

Module 1: Reception and client support

Log sheet	Number to complete	Comments
1a	1	**Reception skills** The SVN has to carry out reception duties, including making appointments, receiving clients and processing payments. The assessor has to complete certain areas (boxes 1, 2 and 3) of the case log identifying key duties observed during reception with reference to the occupational standards.
1b	2	**Admit animals for veterinary procedures** The SVN has to admit two animals for veterinary procedures. Copies of the consent forms should be attached with client details deleted for confidentiality.
1c	2	**Discharge animals after veterinary treatment** The SVN has to discharge two animals following veterinary procedures. These could be cross-referenced to 1b if possible. 1a and 1b should together cover two different types of animal and procedure. At least one (in either 1a or 1b) should be an exotic i.e. not a cat or dog.

		The student should indicate the type of client (i.e. new, current, old, having any special needs) in box 2. One of the cases must include a need for the SVN to demonstrate the administration of medication.
1d	4	**Dispense medication to clients** The SVN should be assessed dispensing POM, PML and GSL drugs to incorporate four different drug classes (e.g. antibiotic, anti-inflammatory), under the direction of a veterinary surgeon. One of these should be a drug that requires special precautions relating to its use e.g. a cytotoxic drug or other potentially hazardous medication. Points to consider, if appropriate include: *Health and safety* *Instructions to the owner not to exceed the stated dose or administer any other medication).* *Dispensing of the drug in a childproof bottle.* *Instruction to the owner regarding storage of the drug.* *Dispensing of a penicillin type drug and the risk of penicillin sensitivity – the client should be instructed to wear gloves.* *Other areas* *Is the owner instructed to give the tablets with or without food?*

If the tablets are required twice daily then the owner should be instructed as to the timing of the doses i.e. equally spaced.

A copy or duplicate of the dispensing label should be included.

These case logs can be cross-referenced to 1c if appropriate.

Calculations should be accurate and have the appropriate units e.g. mg/kg bodyweight.

The duration of the course should correspond to the dates of treatment. If not then an explanation should be given in student comments.

When dispensing flea treatments the owner should be advised to treat the house/dog's bedding etc. They should also be advised to worm their animal against tapeworm. This should all be recorded on the case log. The owner should also be advised to treat any other cats/dogs in the household.

Consistent with the Veterinary Surgeons Act 1966, a veterinary surgeon must prescribe the medication being dispensed. The assessor may sign the log sheet with a statement in the assessor's comments that the drugs dispensed have been prescribed by an identified veterinary surgeon and a statement confirming the student's competence in dispensing the drugs prescribed.

1e	2	**Providing detailed information to clients** The SVN has to give advice to clients on two different occasions, covering two different topics from: *Endoparasitic control – dog or cat* *– two species of parasite* *Ectoparasitic control – dog or cat* *– two species of parasite* *House training (puppy or kitten)* *Oestrus cycle and mating (bitch or queen)* *Euthanasia* *Vaccination (dog or cat)* *Neutering (dog or cat)* *– to include male and female* *Weaning (puppies or kittens)* Points that are relevant but which may not be covered during conversation with the client such as practice policy, underpinning knowledge and alternative approaches should be included in box 4. The assessor may assess these areas through question and answer, in which case a copy of the questions used and answers given should be included and cross-referenced to this section.
1f	1	**Maintain good working relationships with colleagues** Witness statements from assessor and/or suitable witnesses are required to detail how

the SVN conducts him/herself whilst working with other colleagues.

Total number of log sheet for module = 12

NOTE:*Abbreviations e.g. Prescription Only Medicine (POM) should be in full in the first instance. It is then satisfactory to use the abbreviation subsequently in one particular case log. Underpinning knowledge of the above topics may be assessed in the independent assessment (NVQ Level 2 or 3 examinations).*

Module 2: Prepare for and assist with non-surgical veterinary procedures

Log sheet	Number to complete	Comments
2a	5	**Prepare for and assist with non-surgical veterinary procedures** This module must include evidence of dogs, cats and at least one (with a maximum of two) small pets/exotics (i.e. other than cat or dog). A non-surgical procedure should be considered as one that does not require surgical incision and does not normally require a general anaesthetic (unless for restraint). Examples include: *Clinical examination* *Collection of samples for laboratory investigation*

Administration of medication
Application of dressings/bandages
Treatment of wounds
Bathing and cleaning
Examination/cleaning of ears
Administration of fluids
Assisted feeding

Other relevant examples may be included at the discretion of the assessor.

The SVN must provide information on the log sheet regarding the preparation of the environment (e.g. safety and cleanliness), the equipment and materials for the procedure, and the assistance that they provided during the procedure e.g. restraint, raising of a vein etc.

These cases may be cross-referenced to 3b if appropriate.

Total number of log sheets for module = 5

Module 3: Basic nursing

Log sheet	Number to complete	Comments
3a	7	**Basic animal management** Seven cases must be recorded, to include the nursing of dogs, cats and two exotic animals (small pets other than cats or dogs).

Nursing care for a range of veterinary procedures should be covered. Cases that require physiotherapy, basic wound management and hand feeding are possible examples.

Hospitalisation records must be included for two of the cases that detail monitoring and treatment e.g. taking and recording of vital signs, other observations and treatments.

The SVN should demonstrate appropriate feeding of animals, stating the reasons underlying the diet being fed in addition to quantity and frequency. They should also demonstrate appropriate grooming (cleaning, combing and brushing) of the animal during its hospitalisation. Should a particular case not require grooming, the student should detail the reasons for this.

Where there is duplication of information between case logs (e.g. accommodation, bedding, cleaning protocol, ranges for vital signs) the student may consider the use of appendices to which they can refer.

| 3b | 3 | **Basic first aid**
The emphasis on this section should be on basic first aid only. Remember the three aims of first aid are:

1. To preserve life
2. To prevent suffering
3. To prevent the situation deteriorating. |

Therefore, simply applying pressure (via a dry swab/gauze) to prevent further blood loss is basic first aid. Unit 4.4 of the occupational standards provides guidance for this section.

More advanced procedures, such as the placement of indwelling catheters, are not expected.

The first aid event used as evidence can either be in the absence of a veterinary surgeon or assisting the veterinary surgeon (in which case the exact role taken by the SVN should be detailed).

These cases can be cross-referenced to 2a if desired.

The RCVS will currently accept simulated evidence. This should be confirmed, however, with your internal verifier.

3c	5	**Administration of medication** Five cases are required, covering medication administered by the SVN to an animal under the direction of a veterinary surgeon. All administration routes must be covered, i.e. oral, topical, intravenous, subcutaneous and intra-muscular. Calculations should be accurate and have the appropriate units e.g. mg/kg bodyweight.

Health and safety issues may include the need to wear gloves and other protective clothing if required, in addition to comments regarding the need for appropriate restraint of the animal. Where sharps are used, comments should be included regarding their correct disposal. If a controlled drug is used, details of storage and recording requirements are required, in addition to a copy of the register entry if applicable.

These cases should be cross-referenced to other cases in the module where possible.

Total number of log sheets for module = 15

Module 4: Health, safety and security

Log sheet	Number to complete	Comments
4a	1	**Maintain health and safety within the veterinary practice** Record a risk assessment of the animal hospitalisation area, demonstrating a knowledge and understanding of health and safety issues that may arise, how hazards can be minimised and the applicable legislation and regulations. The SVN should be sure to identify all the relevant areas of legislation and ensure that information is accurate and up to date.

		Advice regarding the completion of a risk assessment may be obtained from the person responsible for health and safety within the practice. Alternatively, the Health and Safety Executive can be contacted by telephoning 0541 545500 or by writing to The Health and Safety Executive's Information Centre, Broad Lane, Sheffield S3 7HQ. Information can also be obtained from their website at: www.hse.gov.uk
4b	1	**Respond to human health emergencies (first aid)** One incident of a human health emergency in which the SVN is either directly involved or assists (making their exact role clear). Refer to the three aims of first aid in module 3. The most commonly encountered first aid incident is likely to be an animal bite to the SVN, VN or veterinary surgeon. A photocopy of the accident book entry along with any other requirements of HSE must be included. The assessor may choose to simulate an incident, following discussion with their internal verifier. *OR* Evidence of attendance on a St John's Ambulance/Red Cross first aid course with-

		in the last two years, where competence was assessed, may be used. If so, a copy of the course programme indicating that assessment occurred along with the original certificate should be included. The assessor should include a statement to confirm that he/she is satisfied with the SVN's competence.
4c	1	The SVN should give their account of following security procedures/systems in order to minimise risk to self, others, supplies and equipment (see the occupational standards unit 7, element 3 for guidance). An assessor's statement is required to confirm competence in this area. Security risks should be considered in relation to theft, damage and misuse of drugs and other consumables, equipment, records and personal possessions.

Total number of log sheets for module = 3

10 Guidance notes for modules 5–10 (Edition 2)

Module 5: Laboratory and diagnostic aids

Log sheet	Number to complete	Comments
5a	5	**Laboratory and diagnostic aids** Three different species should be covered in the evidence for this section (dog, cat and small pet/exotic). Two case logs should be completed to include evidence of performance of: 1. Packed cell volume (haematocrit) 2. Blood smear (preparation and staining). This must be of diagnostic quality, but differential counts are not required. Candidates must be able to recognise a good smear and abnormalities as specified in the syllabus. Quantitative results are not required. Two case logs should be completed to include evidence of performance of laboratory procedures involving: 1. Blood biochemistry (to include three tests) 2. Urine 3. Hair/skin 4. Faeces.

		One case log should be completed to include evidence of performance of collection of a specimen for investigation by an outside laboratory. Choice of specimen is optional (but must be different from other specimens used in this module). Emphasis should be placed on the method of collection, storage, preservation and packaging of the specimen. Additional guidance for completion of the log sheets is given in the portfolio itself. All equipment used in each case log must be included.
5b	1	**Maintenance of equipment** One case log should be completed, to include evidence of performance in relation to the maintenance of one piece of laboratory equipment.
5c	1	**Health and safety risk assessment** A risk assessment of the laboratory should be undertaken and recorded to demonstrate a knowledge and understanding of relevant health and safety issues. The SVN should demonstrate their ability to identify and minimise hazards in this area.

Total number of log sheets for module = 7

Module 6: Medical nursing and fluid therapy

Log sheet	Number to complete	Comments
6a	6	**Medical nursing** Three different species should be covered in the evidence for this section (dog, cat and small pet/exotic). Case logs should be completed to include evidence of nursing covering a broad spectrum of medical cases, in which the SVN has played an active role. Cases should be chosen to cover a range of body systems. The SVN should focus upon procedures associated with diagnosis of the condition, administration of treatments and monitoring of the animal. Reference to the occupational standards and syllabus will help in the choice of medical nursing cases. Suggestions include: *Diarrhoeic patients* *Obese patients* *Pregnancy* *Parturition* *Pancreatic insufficiency* *Diabetes mellitus* *Renal failure* *Dermatological conditions* *Cardiac conditions* *Poisoning* *Infectious/contagious diseases*

Expanded case reports

Two of the six medical nursing cases must be expanded to approximately 1000 words and presented as case reports within which the SVN should demonstrate a knowledge and understanding of the condition, treatment and nursing management. A copy of the patient monitoring charts/records must be included as supporting evidence for the two cases. Headings should include:

Case reference
Case details
Presenting problem and history
Preliminary clinical findings
Diagnostic procedures and testing
Treatment and nursing
Ongoing management of the condition
Outcome and case evaluation

| 6b | 3 | **Fluid therapy** |

Three case logs should be completed to include evidence of performance in relation to the administration of fluid therapy. The SVN should have played an active role in the administration and maintenance of fluid therapy and monitoring of the animal, and should have placed an intravenous catheter on at least one of the occasions. This should be made clear in the case log sheet(s). A copy of the patient monitoring chart used to record and monitor fluid therapy should be included for each case log.

A cat and a dog should be included, as should three of the following types of fluid therapy:

1. Crystalloids
2. Colloids
3. Blood
4. Oral re-hydration.

These should be cross-referenced wherever possible to the medical nursing case logs in 6a. Other cross-referencing may also be used.

*Total number of log sheets for module = 9
plus 2 expanded reports*

Module 7: Radiography

Log sheet	Number to complete	Comments
7a	9	**Radiography** Three different species should be covered in this section (dog, cat and small pet/exotic). Nine case logs should be completed to include evidence of performance of different radiographic procedures in which the candidate has played a central role, covering a broad range of procedures/positioning. The objective standards and syllabus will help in the choice of cases. One procedure must include the use of contrast media. Radiographic projections may be selected from the following; other standard projections may be used.

		Shoulder lateral/caudocranial *Elbow lateral/craniocaudal* *Carpus lateral/dorsopalmar* *Stifle lateral/caudocranial* *Hock* lateral/craniocaudal* *Phalanges (forelimb) dorsoplantar* *Phalanges (hindlimb) dorsoplantar* *Abdomen lateral/ventrodorsal* *Thorax lateral/dorsoventral or ventrodorsal* *Pelvis lateral/ventrodorsal* *Pelvis for submission to British Veterinary Association/Kennel Club Hip Dysplasia Scheme* *Skull lateral/dorsoventral* *Intra-oral* *Cervical spine lateral/ventrodorsal* *Thoracic spine lateral/ventrodorsal* *Lumbar spine lateral/ventrodorsal* *Hock position should be dorsoplantar (craniocaudal applies *above* the hock). Only one view should be used per log sheet.
7b	1	**Health and safety risk assessment** A risk assessment of the X-ray room should be undertaken and recorded to demonstrate a knowledge and understanding of relevant health and safety issues. The SVN should demonstrate ability to identify and minimise hazards during radiographic procedures.

Total number of log sheets for module = 10

Module 8: Surgical nursing and theatre practice

Log sheet	Number to complete	Comments
8a	1	**Surgical nursing and theatre practice** Three different species should be covered in the evidence for this section (dog, cat and small pet/exotic). **Maintain asepsis** One case log should be completed to include evidence of how the SVN prepares and maintains the surgical theatre to contribute towards the maintenance of asepsis.
8b	2	**Sterilisation** Two case logs should be completed to include evidence of the SVN's performance of two sterilisation techniques, one of which must be sterilisation by autoclave.
8c	6	**Preparation and assisting – surgical procedures** Three different species should be covered in the evidence for this section (dog, cat and small pet/exotic). At least one case must include a dressing or bandage that the SVN has applied, with details and reasons for the materials selected.

The SVN is expected to provide aseptic surgical assistance (under instruction from the veterinary surgeon) on at least one occasion. This should be detailed in the case log sheet.

Appendices should be used for procedures that are standard across all cases; however, they must be clearly referenced and signed by both the SVN and the assessor.

Six case logs should be completed, to include evidence of involvement of the SVN in the nursing management of six surgical procedures. The candidate must demonstrate competence in:

1. The selection and preparation of surgical equipment and materials
2. The preparation of animals for surgical procedures
3. Assisting the veterinary surgeon during surgical procedures
4. Assisting the recovery of animals after surgical procedures.

Cases should be selected to cover a broad range of surgical procedures and reflect a number of body systems. Reference to the objective syllabus/occupational standards may help in the choice of cases for assessment.

Further guidance on completion of the case

log sheets is included in the module guidance notes of the portfolio.

Expanded case reports

Two of the six surgical cases must be expanded to approximately 1000 words and presented as case reports within which the SVN should demonstrate a knowledge and understanding of the condition, treatment and nursing management. A copy of the patient monitoring records should be included for each case. Headings should include:

Case reference
Case details
History and diagnosis
The surgical procedure
Recovery and postoperative nursing
Outcome and case evaluation

8d	3	**Maintenance of equipment**

Maintenance of equipment

Three case logs should be completed, to include evidence of performance of the SVN's ability to monitor and maintain equipment associated with surgical procedures. They must demonstrate to the assessor that they can prepare equipment for use, clean and sterilise it and identify and report any malfunction.

The three assessments should cover three pieces of equipment from the following:

ECG
Endoscope
Cryosurgical equipment
Diathermy/electrosurgery
Electric clippers
Ventilator
Suction pump
Powered dental equipment
Powered drill

Total number of log sheets for module = 12
plus 2 expanded case reports

Module 9: Anaesthesia

Log sheet	*Number to complete*	*Comments*
9a	6	**Anaesthesia record** Three different species should be covered in the evidence for this section (dog, cat and small pet/exotic). The cases should be chosen to cover a range of equipment, circuits, drugs and gases used in the practice. Six case logs should be completed, to include evidence of active involvement of the SVN. The SVN must be competent in: 1. The preparation of equipment, drugs and other supplies

		2. Assistance with the anaesthetic procedure and recovery of the animal.
9b	1	**Health and safety risk assessment** A risk assessment of the X-ray operating theatre should be undertaken, with the emphasis on the use of anaesthetic equipment, gases, drugs and activities associated with anaesthesia. It should demonstrate a knowledge and understanding of relevant health and safety issues, and the ability to identify and minimise hazards in this area during anaesthesia.
9c	1	**Anaesthetic emergency box** The SVN must record the contents of the emergency box on the log sheet, giving details of the circumstances under which each drug/piece of equipment would be used. The SVN must also give a brief account of an occasion when they were required to provide equipment from the emergency box in relation to a case in which they were involved. If this situation does not occur naturally then simulation and questioning by the assessor can be used. Any questions and answers given by the SVN should be recorded and included as evidence.

Total number of log sheets for module = 8

Module 10: Maintain the availability of veterinary resources

Log sheet	Number to complete	Comments
10a	1	**Maintain the supply of veterinary materials** There may be the option within this module to cross-reference evidence from other areas of the portfolio. If this is the case, the log sheet reference number, page number and box number of the evidence should be written in the appropriate box(es) on the log sheet. It should be remembered that evidence completed in this way must cover all aspects and be current.

One case log should be completed, to include evidence of the SVN placing a small order (one or more items) with a wholesaler or other supplier.

Items should be chosen from the following:

Medications
Drugs
Documentation
Equipment
Sterile supplies
Consumables e.g. pet foods/dietary products

A photocopy of the order form must be attached to the log sheet. |

10b	1	**Maintain the availability of veterinary equipment** One case log should be completed, to include evidence of the SVN's maintenance of the availability of equipment for use in the veterinary practice.
10c	1	**Maintain the availability of veterinary examination rooms** One case log should be completed by a suitable witness regarding the SVN's competence in the maintenance of examination rooms within the veterinary practice. Discussion with the assessor will be required as to the suitability of any witness.

Total number of log sheets for module = 3

11 Portfolio submission and outcomes

If a student is working for a Training Practice (TP) then their portfolio should be submitted to the VNAC once complete. Guidance should be sought from the VNAC regarding its submission procedure and any deadline dates and fees that may have been established.

If submitting directly to the RCVS (if the practice is still an ATAC) guidelines for the submission of the veterinary nurse portfolio are issued and these should always be confirmed prior to submission. At the time of publication the RCVS guidelines can be summarised as set out below.

Before submission of the relevant modules of the portfolio, special attention should be made to check the following:

- That all log sheets are completed in full and signed by both the SVN and assessor.
- That the authentication sheet in the portfolio lists all the signatures that appear in the portfolio, with the designation of each individual being clearly documented.
- That all evidence that could identify a client, by name, address or any other means recognisable outside the veterinary practice, has been removed from the case logs and any supporting evidence.
- That all pages are numbered in the bottom right hand corner and a contents list is enclosed in the front of the portfolio.
- That a hard copy of the entire submission is retained by the SVN. A copy on computer disk is inappropriate, as this will not have the relevant signatures and assessor comments.

The following items must be submitted for external verification (if the practice is not a VNAC or TP):

- A submission form with the appropriate sections completed by the SVN and the Practice Principal.
- The personal profile and details of college-based training.
- The authentication sheet (fully completed).
- The action plan for the relevant level of S/NVQ.
- The case log sheets and any essential supporting evidence for the relevant modules.
- A contents list indexing all submitted papers.

If any of the above are omitted, the RCVS may return the portfolio as unsatisfactory and it will need to be submitted when complete.

The following items should not be submitted:

- Portfolio folder.
- Log sheets for modules that are not appropriate to the particular level (these will differ depending upon the edition of the portfolio).
- Module instructions.
- Commercially produced leaflets.
- Items that are not essential for the portfolio evidence.

11.1 Submission procedures

If a student is working for a Training Practice (TP) then their portfolio should be submitted to the VNAC once complete. Guidance should be sought from the VNAC regarding its submission procedure and any deadline dates and fees that may have been established.

If submitting directly to the RCVS as an ATAC, the submission sheets should be completed using black ink and capital letters. The return address for the portfolio should be completed.

All the relevant items discussed above should be included and placed in the following order:

1. Submissions sheet
2. Contents list
3. Personal profile sheets
4. Authentication sheet
5. Action plan
6. Case log sheets.

A copy of the entire submission should be kept.

Plastic wallets/pockets should NOT be submitted. Reinforcing rings should be used to strengthen the holes in any sheets, where necessary.

The items above should be secured with treasury tags, placed in a strong envelope and posted to:

The Royal College of Veterinary Surgeons
Belgravia House
62–64 Horseferry Road
London
SW1P 2AF

Recorded delivery is recommended for posting and the SVN is advised to maintain the receipt as proof of posting until the portfolio is returned.

The portfolio may be delivered in person to Belgravia House between 9am and 4pm, Monday to Friday.

The RCVS considers the portfolio to be the responsibility of the SVN until it reaches the RCVS, and does not recommend any other means of delivery other than those above.

Five working days should be allowed for the portfolio to reach the RCVS and this should be taken into consideration when posting close to the submission deadline. Proof of posting is not considered sufficient evidence should the portfolio fail to meet the submission deadline.

Great care should be taken to establish whether the SVN is required to submit their portfolio to the RCVS or a VNAC (the latter will only be applicable if the practice is approved as a VNAC or TP).

11.2 Return of the portfolio

If a student is working for a Training Practice (TP) then their portfolio should be submitted to the VNAC once complete. Guidance should be sought from the VNAC regarding its timescale for verification and return. A copy of the IV's report will be sent to the assessor once the portfolio has been internally verified. It may be a requirement that the VNAC retains the student portfolio for external verification by the RCVS. It should be remembered that, technically, all portfolios could be subject to external verification by the RCVS; however, it is likely that the external verifier will choose a random sample to verify.

If the portfolio is submitted directly to the RCVS, as the practice is still of ATAC status, then the RCVS aim to have the portfolio returned within six weeks following submission. During busy periods, for example near the submission deadline, they recognise that this period may extend to eight weeks. The returned portfolio also has the following accompanying documents:

- A copy of the submission form with a report from the external verifier (EV), indicating whether or not the portfolio contains sufficient evidence to meet the national standards
- A letter explaining the outcome and any action that may be necessary.
- A sealed envelope which contains a second copy of the EV's report which should be treated as confidential and given to the assessor. The assessor may then discuss any relevant issues with the SVN.

If still an ATAC, the Practice Principal is informed of the outcome of external verification and is sent the EV's report to highlight any action required by the assessor.

11.3 Portfolio submissions and outcomes for practices with VNAC or TP approval

The VNAC will confirm with the practice the procedure for portfolio submission and internal verification. In most cases, portfolios will be requested at two stages for internal verification – once during an interim period prior to completion and again for internal verification once the portfolio is complete. The student should follow the VNAC guidelines for portfolio submission. Once complete, the VNAC may be required to retain a number of portfolios for external verification by the RCVS. The VNAC should inform the TP if this is the case. The assessor will be informed in writing of the outcome of the internal verification process by the VNAC.

12 Terminology

Although every effort has been made to make this publication free of the 'jargon' that is commonly associated with S/NVQs, it is necessary that all those involved with the S/NVQ are familiar with appropriate terminology. For clarity and ease of reference, a list of relevant terms and abbreviations is provided below.

Accreditation
The formal act by which the Qualification Curriculum Authority recognises statements of competence and approves awarding bodies and their qualifications for inclusion in the S/NVQ framework.

Area of competence
A sub-division of the total occupational field to which a set of S/NVQs relates.

Assessment
The process of collecting evidence and making judgements on whether performance criteria have been met.

Assessor
The person responsible for checking that the level required for skills, knowledge and understanding has been achieved. (A listed veterinary nurse or veterinary surgeon who holds the appropriate assessor units.)

ATAC
Approved Training and Assessment Centre. Formerly known as an ATC, an Approved Training Centre. Veterinary practices that were approved as ATCs in the past by the RCVS will

have to go through a re-approval process to train veterinary nurses towards the S/NVQs.

Award
A general term for that which is given to an individual for the attainment of an S/NVQ.

Awarding body
The RCVS is a body approved by the Qualification Curriculum Authority for the purpose of awarding S/NVQs in veterinary nursing.

Candidate
An individual undertaking an S/NVQ.

Certificate
A document issued to an individual by an awarding body, formally attesting to the attainment of an S/NVQ or a unit of competence.

Competence
The ability to perform in work roles or jobs to the standards required in employment.

Evidence gatherer
A qualified veterinary surgeon or listed veterinary nurse who does not hold a TDLB qualification in assessment but may act as an assessor. All evidence assessed by an evidence gatherer is subject to assessment by a TDLB assessor and verification by an internal verifier.

External verifier
A person appointed by the awarding body, the RCVS, who is

responsible for checking and monitoring assessments carried out in VNACs.

Internal verifier

A person holding the appropriate internal verifier qualification who checks that assessments are carried out fairly, consistently and to the standard required by the awarding body – in this case the RCVS.

Lead (or standard-setting) body

A body responsible for the specification of standards of competence, made up of representatives of employers, employees and professions, and their advisers, as appropriate.

Lead Body

The Veterinary Lead Body, who are responsible for creating the national standards for the veterinary nurse industry upon which the VN qualification is based.

Level

A sub-division of the S/NVQ framework which is used to define progressive degrees of competence.

NVQ

National Vocational Qualification, an award based upon occupational standards, offered in England, Wales and Northern Ireland.

NVQ criteria

The principles with which qualifications and their awarding bodies must conform for their accreditation and recognition by the QCA.

NVQ framework
The national system for ordering NVQs according to levels and areas of competence.

Occupation
The collective term for jobs in an area of employment which require common aspects of competence.

Occupational standards
'Guidelines to the practice to which students are assessed' – details of which are in the RCVS Training Centre Handbook.

Performance criteria
The criteria which indicate the standard of performance required for the successful achievement of an element of competence.

QCA
Qualifications Curriculum Authority, the accrediting body for NVQs in England, Wales and Northern Ireland. The QCA is responsible for accrediting NVQs in all areas and for auditing every awarding body to check that appropriate systems are in place and are being implemented effectively.

RCVS
The Royal College of Veterinary Surgeons, awarding body for the Veterinary Nursing S/NVQs.

SQA
Scottish Qualifications Authority, the accrediting body for SVQs in Scotland. The responsibilities of the SQA are similar to those of the QCA.

Standard of competence
The specification of competence for employment upon which a NVQ is based, stated in the form of title, units, elements and performance criteria.

Standard of performance
The measure of performance required for the achievement of an element of competence as indicated by the related performance criteria.

SVN
A student veterinary nurse, also known as a candidate when working towards the veterinary nursing S/NVQ.

SVQ
Scottish Vocational Qualification, an award based upon occupational standards, offered in Scotland.

TP
Training Practice (see Appendix A).

Unit of competence
A primary sub-division of the competence required for the award of an NVQ, representing a discrete aspect of competence having meaning in employment which may be recognised and certificated independently as a credit towards an award. A unit is made up of elements of competence.

VNAC
Veterinary Nurse Approved Centre (see Appendix A).

Example case log sheets for modules 1–4

LOG SHEET 1A: RECEPTION SKILLS

Student Veterinary Nurse's Name:	VN Enrolment No:
A Nonymous	1234

NB: Boxes 1, 2 & 3 to be completed by the Assessor
(or suitable Witness or Evidence Gatherer)

1. Date and location of surgery/clinic session:

26 October 2001 at Any Vet Veterinary Hospital – Morning Surgery

2. Duration of reception duties:

Time of surgery start: 9am
Time of surgery finish: 11am

3. Details of reception duties and procedures dealt with:

I observed Anna dealing with the following duties and procedures:

- Greeting clients with their animals for appointments.
- Making appointments with clients in person and over the telephone.
- Dealing with queries regarding surgery times and house visits.
- Processing payments by cash, cheque and Switch/Visa.
- Prioritising an emergency case that arrived unexpectedly.
- Giving advice about veterinary treatments and procedures.
- Dealing with an aggressive dog in the reception area.

During this time she dealt with current, new, young and old clients.

Student's Comments:
to include any difficulties or unusual requirements and reflective comment

Reception is always very busy during morning surgery, however I always try to remain calm and greet the clients in a pleasant manner. Some clients can become difficult at times, however I always try to deal with this in a professional manner.

Assessor's Statement:

The student has been observed carrying out reception duties during the surgery session as specified. Competence has been demonstrated in accordance with our practice policy and the relevant occupational standards.

Comments:
Anna is competent when carrying out reception duties and is able to deal with most situations that arise. I have questioned her to cover those areas not evident from

performance (recorded in Appendix A) and am happy that she meets the national standard as detailed in Unit 1, elements 1.1, 1.2, 1.3 and 1.4.

Assessor's Signature: Date:

Assessor's Name: Assessor's Qualifications:

LOG SHEET 1B: ADMIT ANIMALS FOR VETERINARY TREATMENT

Student Veterinary Nurse's Name: A Nonymous	VN Enrolment No: 1234

1. Case number-identification:

RCS 1

2. Case details:

Species: Canine	*Breed:* Boxer	*Client Type:* Current
Sex: Female (Entire)	*Age:* 2yrs 6mths	*Weight:* 26kg

3. Reason for admission ie. procedure:

General anaesthesia and ovario-hysterectomy

4. Date and time animal admitted:

26th October 2001 8.50am

5. Date animal discharged:

26th October 2001

6. Information given to client when admitted:

I confirmed with the client that:

- The animal had been fasted for 12 hours.
- The animal had been given the opportunity to urinate and defecate that morning.
- Water had been withheld that morning.
- The client understood the planned procedure.

The consent form was explained and then signed by the client. I advised the client that the procedure was planned for the morning operating session and that they should telephone the surgery at 2pm for a progress report.

7. Action taken by student on admission of the animal:

I ensured the animal's details were correct and completed the hospitalisation record.

I removed the client's own collar and lead which was labelled and put on to the animal's hook in the ward along with the signed consent form.

I placed a slip lead onto the animal and took it from the consulting room into the ward, where it was weighed and then placed in an appropriate kennel with the animal's hospital record attached to the front of the kennel. The animal's details were then entered on to the hospital board.

I monitored and recorded the animal's temperature, pulse and respiration rate. The animal was then left in the kennel until the veterinary surgeon was ready to examine it and administer the premedication.

Student's Comments and Signature:

When I am involved with admitting animals I always try to be reassuring to the client who is often anxious about leaving their pet. I think that this is a very important role for a student or qualified veterinary nurse.

The evidence in this log sheet is a true representation of my involvement in the case described, and the work undertaken in compiling the log is my own.

Student Veterinary Nurse's Signature:

Assessor's Statement:

The procedures and details associated with the admission procedure described have been observed by me and have been carried out correctly and competently.

Comments:

During the direct observation of Anna admitting this patient, she proved to be competent. It was also evident during further verbal questioning (see Appendix A) that she had a good level of knowledge in this area, relating to the occupational standards.

Assessor's Signature: *Date:*

Assessor's Name: *Assessor's Qualifications:*

LOG SHEET 1C: DISCHARGE ANIMALS AFTER VETERINARY TREATMENT

Student Veterinary Nurse's Name:	VN Enrolment No:
A Nonymous	1234

1. Case number-identification:

RCS 3

2. Case details:

Species: Canine	*Breed:* Boxer	*Client Type:* Current
Sex: Female (Entire)	*Age:* 2yrs 6mths	*Weight:* 26kg

3. Veterinary procedure carried out:

General anaesthesia and ovario-hysterectomy

4. Date and time animal discharged:

26th October 2001

5. Date and time of next appointment:

31st October 2001

6. Describe any preparation of the animal prior to discharge:

Prior to discharge the patient was groomed and the surgical site was checked. There was a small amount of dry blood on the skin that was gently cleaned away using cotton wool and a 2% solution of Hibiscrub. The injection site on the right forelimb was also checked but did not need further attention as it was clean.

7. Information and advice given to the client:

The client was given the following information verbally:

- Keep Millie warm and in a quiet area this evening.
- No exercise this evening, however allow her to go in to the garden to urinate and defecate.
- Offer a small amount of bland food this evening e.g. chicken or white fish with boiled rice.
- The sutures are non-absorbable and will require removal in 10 days, until which time she should be exercised only on a lead for short periods of time e.g. 10min 4 times daily.
- Millie should be brought back to the surgery after 5 days to be checked by the veterinary surgeon.

- If Millie displays any unusual signs (e.g. vomiting, off food, unable to settle), contact the surgery for advice.
- If Millie starts to lick or chew the sutures, the Elizabethan collar should be put on to prevent further interference.

This information is also provided in the postoperative care sheet that was given to the owner.

8. State any medication or treatment(s) supplied to the owner:*

Rimadyl (Carporphen) 50mg x 6. Refer to RSC 5

* Details can be cross-referenced to dispensing logs.

9. Was the method for administering any medication or treatment(s) to the animal demonstrated to the owner?

☐ *YES*   ☐ *NO*

Comment:
I gave a demonstration how to safely administer the tablets. Refer to RSC 5

Student's Comments and Signature:

When discharging Millie I initially explained everything to the owner prior to bringing Millie from the ward. I feel that this is important because many owners are more interested in fussing their pet and do not listen to the postoperative care of the patient.

The evidence in this log sheet is a true representation of my involvement in the case described, and the work undertaken in compiling the log is my own.

Student Veterinary Nurse's Signature:

Assessor's Statement:

The procedures and details associated with the discharge procedure described have been observed by me and have been carried out correctly and competently.

Comments:
I observed Anna whilst she was discussing aftercare with this client and she demonstrated a good understanding of the subject and maintained a professional but friendly manner with the client. I feel that she is competent in this area.

Assessor's Signature: *Date:*

Assessor's Name: *Assessor's Qualifications:*

LOG SHEET 1D: DISPENSING MEDICATION TO CLIENTS

Student Veterinary Nurse's Name:	VN Enrolment No:
A Nonymous	1234

1. Case number-identification:

RCS 5

2. Case details:

Species: Canine	*Breed:* Boxer	*Client Type:* Current
Sex: Female (Entire)	*Age:* 2yrs 6mths	*Weight:* 26kg

3. Name of drug dispensed (to include trade and generic names):

Trade name: Rimadyl (50mg)
Generic name: Carprofen

4. Legal dispensing category and drug classification:

Dispensing category: Prescription Only Medicine (POM)
Prescribing Group: Non-steroidal anti-inflammatory

5. Dose given (include calculations):

Dose rate: 2mg/kg bodyweight, twice daily (b.i.d.) for 3 days

Dose given (including calculation): 2 x 26 = 52mg twice daily

Each tablet is 50mg, therefore 1 tablet twice daily for three days dispensed
i.e. 6 tablets in total.

6. Reason for administration and route:

Reason: to act as pain relief, postoperatively, following an ovario-hysterectomy.
Route: Orally, as the drug is effective via this route and easily administered by the owner.

7. Health & Safety, and other dispensing notes: *to include a duplicate or copy of the dispensing label and Health and Safety issues*

- Client instructed to give tablets at evenly spaced intervals (am and pm).
- Can be given with or without food at owner's preference.
- Client advised to keep the tablets out of reach of children and the drug was dispensed in a childproof container.

A printed label should be included here as evidence of the drug dispensed.

8. Additional advice/instructions given to client:

State how you ensured the client was able to administer the medication/treatment and any other information provided.

The client asked how to administer the tablets, so I described the technique and demonstrated for them. They were not sure whether they would be able to do this so I advised that they purchase a small packet of "pill poppas" (small treats) to hide the tablet in when giving to Millie. Most clients find these very useful, however I did warn them to observe Millie to check that the tablet had been swallowed, as some dogs have the ability to eat the treat and not the tablet. If they continued to have trouble, I advised them to bring her down to the surgery where I could administer the tablet for them.

9. Date of dispensing:

26.10.01

10. Briefly state the procedure carried out by you, when processing payment for the items dispensed (if applicable):

The clients settled their account by Switch card. I checked the date on the card and processed the payment through the machine. After checking the amount on the slip I asked them to sign the slip and checked the signature with that on the back of the card.

Student's Comments and Signature:

I dispense medicine, under the direction of a veterinary surgeon, to clients on a regular basis and am confident that I can deal with any of their questions regarding administration of medication. In this case, the owner had no problems in convincing Millie to eat the tablet hidden in the "pill poppa".

The evidence in this log sheet is a true representation of my involvement in the case described, and the work undertaken in compiling the log is my own.

Student Veterinary Nurse's Signature:

Assessor's Statement:

The procedures and details associated with the dispensing record described have been observed by me and have been carried out correctly and competently.

Comments:
Anna dispensed the medication under the direction of our veterinary surgeon, Mr Small. Questioning confirmed that she is aware of the legal dispensing categories and the implications for dispensing to clients (see Appendix A).

Assessor's Signature: *Date:*

Assessor's Name: *Assessor's Qualifications:*

LOG SHEET 1E: DETAILED CLIENT INFORMATION

Student Veterinary Nurse's Name:	VN Enrolment No:
A Nonymous	1234

1. Subject discussed with owner:

Ovario-hysterectomy

2. Briefly state the circumstances in which you were required to provide information on this subject: *to include client type e.g. new, current, young, old, having any special needs*

This was a new client, who has recently acquired a collie cross bitch. The client is middle-aged with no apparent special needs.

Date information given: 10.10.01

3. Your account of the specific information given:

I gave the following advice to the client regarding having her bitch neutered:

- The veterinary surgeon in this practice recommends that spaying is performed prior to the first season for the following reasons:
  1. The uterus is generally much smaller which makes the procedure easier.
  2. There is a lower incidence of mammary tumour development in bitches spayed before their first season.
  3. There is no evidence that allowing a normal sized dog to have a season is beneficial.
- I explained that the procedure is a routine one that is performed regularly, however, there is always a slight risk with anaesthetics and surgical procedures.
- I discussed the benefits of spaying which included:
  1. No unwanted pregnancies.
  2. No seasons.
  3. Less likely to roam or attract males.
  4. Removal of the risk of conditions affecting the upper genital tract e.g. pyometra.
- I also discussed the possible disadvantages of spaying which were:
  1. Weight gain due to reduced metabolism.
  2. Change in coat texture/condition.
  3. Acquired sphincter mechanism incompetence in later life causing urinary incontinence.
  4. Behavioural changes.
- I explained that generally:
  - Patients were dropped off early in the morning.
  - Surgery would be performed that day.
  - Providing that there were no complications she would go home that evening.
  - She would be checked by a vet 5 days post surgery.
  - Sutures would be removed by a nurse 10 days post surgery.

4. Additional information (or expansion) on the subject not covered in your discussion:

The following information was not discussed, however, it would be explained when the client made an appointment for surgery and at the discharge appointment respectively:

- Esme would need to be starved prior to the procedure i.e. nothing to eat after 8pm the previous night.
- Water should be withheld from 6am on the morning of the operation.
- An appointment would be made to admit Esme when you could ask further questions if necessary.
- Esme would need to go for a walk prior to admission so that she could empty her bowels and bladder.

And

- On going home she should be allowed to sleep in a warm, quiet area.
- She should not be allowed to play, run or jump e.g. no climbing stairs.
- She must only have lead exercise for the two weeks following surgery.
- The evening of the operation she will need a light diet which will be given to you before leaving the surgery.
- You will be given an Elizabethan collar that must be put on if she shows signs of licking or chewing the incision.

Student's Comments and Signature: *to include details of how easy you found it to convey the advice verbally to the owner(s)*

I enjoy giving clients advice because part of being a good nurse is having good communication skills, it also makes clients aware that nurses play an important role in the veterinary practice.

The evidence in this log sheet is a true representation of my involvement in the case described, and the work undertaken in compiling the log is my own.

Student Veterinary Nurse's Signature:

Assessor's Statement:

The advice and information included in this log sheet has been conveyed to the client(s) by the student – this has been observed by me and I consider it to have been carried out both correctly and effectively. Additional information provided (box 4) is correct and sufficient.

Comments:

Anna gave extensive information to this client. She also was aware of other information that needed to be given but was not relevant at the time. She has displayed good underpinning knowledge.

Assessor's Signature: *Date:*

Assessor's Name: *Assessor's Qualifications:*

LOG SHEET 1F: ASSESSOR'S STATEMENT
Maintain good working relationships with colleagues

Student Veterinary Nurse's Name:	VN Enrolment No:
A Nonymous	1234

1. Colleagues:

Please provide comments about how the student relates to colleagues in order to maintain good working relationships within the veterinary practice.

Anna has a very good working relationship with all members of staff and always tries her hardest to get on with everyone, even when others can be difficult at times.

Witness' Name: *Date:*

2. Providing information:

Please confirm that the student provides clear and accurate information to colleagues on request and at appropriate opportunities.
I can confirm that Anna always provides clear, accurate information when requested.

Example of information and circumstances:
- Information about clients in circumstances when difficulties/disputes have occurred.
- Information about animals to other nurses and veterinary surgeons.
- information to colleagues about reasons for absence from work.

Witness' Name: *Date:*

3. Carrying out requests:

Please confirm the student responds promptly to requests from colleagues, ensuring work can be carried out efficiently.
I can confirm that Anna is always helpful and will do her best to ensure requests from colleagues are completed.

Example of request and area of work:
Requests to cover reception due to staff illness, requests to break from usual routine to help others, request to clean areas that others may have overlooked.

Please confirm that the student refers to the appropriate person when experiencing difficulties with requests.
If Anna experiences any problems she always refers back to inform them of the problem and request help and advice.

Witness' Name: *Date:*

Student Veterinary Nurse's Signature:

Assessor's Statement:

Sufficient and reliable evidence has been presented to confirm the student can maintain good working relationships with colleagues.

Comments:

Anna is a valued member of staff who is a popular member of her practice team due to her friendly and helpful manner. She is aware of the difficulties that are sometimes encountered within our practice and knows how to deal with them and who to go to for help and advice.

Assessor's Signature: *Date:*

Assessor's Name: *Assessor's Qualifications:*

LOG SHEET 2A: PREPARE AND ASSIST FOR VETERINARY NON-SURGICAL PROCEDURES

Student Veterinary Nurse's Name:	VN Enrolment No:
A Nonymous	1234

1. Procedure prepared for:

Application of a Robert Jones Bandage

2. Date:

26th October 2001

3. Type of animal:

Species: Canine   *Breed:* Staffordshire Bull Terrier

Sex: Male (Entire)   *Age:* 6yrs   *Weight:* 23kg

4. Preparation of the environment in which the procedure takes place:

The prep room was tidied and the table on which Bruce was going to be placed was cleaned with Trigene disinfectant (1:100). The work surfaces were cleaned with this solution.

5. Preparation of the equipment and materials:

The following equipment was prepared:

- Lister bandage scissors
- Roll of cotton wool
- 4 cohesive conforming bandages 5cm e.g. Easifix Cohesive Smith+Nephew
- 2 cohesive conforming bandages 7.5cm e.g. Coplus Smith+Nephew
- 2.5cm Elastoplast for stirrups
- Empty drip bag to protect the distal portion of the bandage.

6. Assisting with the procedure:

Describe briefly:

a. *How the animal was prepared, handled and restrained.*

b. *State if any additional information was necessary in order to assist with the procedure, e.g. previous records, instruction manuals/reference material.*

c. *Any other details about your role in assisting with the procedure.*

Bruce was lifted onto the examination table by myself and another nurse. I followed the correct lifting procedure, keeping my back straight, bending my knees and having my feet hip distance apart.

I was holding the front of the patient and in order to lay him on the table my colleague and I took the animal's legs away from us while we also supported his head and body. Once he was laid on the table I placed one arm over his neck to prevent him from banging his head and injuring himself. I used the same hand to hold his underneath limb. My other hand held his other forelimb. The other nurse held one hind limb in each hand and applied gentle pressure on his body to prevent him from struggling. When the qualified veterinary nurse was ready to apply the bandage, I used both of my hands to hold the affected limb (upper forelimb), keeping it as straight and still as possible.

During the procedure I talked to Bruce to offer him reassurance.

When the procedure was completed we lifted him down from the table and I walked him back to his kennel.

Student's Comments and Signature:

It is important to be confident and firm when handling and restraining animals. This helps to prevent any injuries to the handler, the patient or those involved in administering veterinary care. It also makes the procedure easier and less time consuming.

The evidence in this log sheet is a true representation of my involvement in the case described, and the work undertaken in compiling the log is my own.

Student Veterinary Nurse's Signature:

Assessor's Statement:

The procedures and details described have been observed by me and have been carried out correctly and competently.

Comments:

I observed Anna while she restrained this patient and she proved to have good practical skills. Questioning revealed a good underpinning knowledge (see Appendix A).

_____

Assessor's Signature: *Date:*

_____

Assessor's Name: *Assessor's Qualifications:*

LOG SHEET 3A: BASIC ANIMAL MANAGEMENT

Student Veterinary Nurse's Name:	VN Enrolment No:
A Nonymous	1234

1. Case number-identification:

BN1

2. Case details:

Species: Canine　　　*Breed:* Shetland Sheep Dog

Sex: Female (Entire)　　*Age:* 13yrs　　　*Weight:* 10.8kg

3. Reason for hospitalisation:

Hospitalised following surgical removal of an extensive mixed mammary tumour, left caudal abdominal gland. Hospitalisation allowed the wound to be monitored in the initial postoperative period whilst the patient recovered fully from general anaesthesia.

4. Type of accommodation and bedding material used:
to include any relevant environmental factors

Kennel:　　　　　Width 60cm, depth 90cm, height 60cm.
Construction:　　Tiled breeze block walls, tiled floor, steel mesh door, locker-type kennels.
Bedding:　　　　Newspaper and a blanket.
Environment:　　Temperature in kennel block regulated by a thermostat set at 20°C. Noise kept to a minimum by isolating noisy dogs in separate kennel area...
　　　　　　　　Radio playing at low level for reassurance for animals.
　　　　　　　　Ventilation regulated by manually operated extractor fans removing stale air and odours, minimising the risk of airborne infection.

5. Accommodation cleaning protocol: to include type of disinfectant, dilution of, mechanical cleaning procedures, frequency of cleaning, disposal of waste

After the bitch had stayed in overnight, her kennel had not been soiled. She was put in an outside run where she passed urine. Her blanket and paper were removed and the kennel brushed out to remove fluff and hair. A fresh blanket and paper were then put in before she was brought back from the run. After she had been discharged her kennel was completely cleaned as per the cleaning protocol on Appendix 1.

6. Feeding regime:

The patient was initially starved, with water available in small quantities during the evening after surgery, once she had returned to full consciousness. On the morning following surgery she was offered a small quantity (2 tablespoons) of Waltham canine selected protein. This is an easily digestible palatable diet that helps to ensure adequate nutrition, especially protein intake, after surgery in order to compensate for the increase in metabolic rate that occurs. A further meal of 1/4 of 100g can of canine selected protein was offered later that day (1pm), which she ate, before being returned to her owner.

7. Nursing care and monitoring of the animal: *Give details of grooming, wound management, cleaning, monitoring of vital signs and TLC*

Postoperatively the wound was gently cleaned to remove any trickles of blood around the surgical site. Any contamination of hairs around the shaved area was washed off. Observations of Sasha's vital signs (temperature, pulse and respiration) were monitored and were within normal ranges (see Appendix 1 for normal ranges in the dog).

The following day her temperature, pulse and respiration rate were checked (again within normal ranges). The wound was checked and needed no further cleaning. Sasha's eyes, nose, anus and vulva were checked for discharge and her eyes were cleaned. Her coat was gently brushed with a slicker brush to remove knots and tangles. During this time I talked to Sasha to provide her with stimulation and company.

8. Medication administered: *details can be cross-referenced to Log 3c*

The veterinary surgeon decided not to administer any medication in this case.

9. Date(s): *specify duration of hospitalisation*

29.10.01 Admission, surgery and postoperative hospitalisation overnight
30.10.01 Hospitalised until 3pm when discharged to owner

Student's Comments: *to include the part the student has played in this case*

Copy of hospitalisation record attached. ☑ *YES* ☐ *NO*
There were no complications with Sasha during her stay, during which I had sole responsibility for her nursing care.
The evidence in this log sheet is a true representation of my involvement in the case described, and the work undertaken in compiling the log is my own.
Student Veterinary Nurse's Signature:

Assessor's Statement:

The procedures and details associated with the basic animal management described have been observed by me and have been carried out correctly and competently.

Comments:
Anna has a good understanding of nursing procedures relating to hospitalised clients. On questioning she was able to explain the importance of such procedures (see Appendix A).

Assessor's Signature:	*Date:*

Assessor's Name:	*Assessor's Qualifications:*

LOG SHEET 3B: BASIC FIRST AID

Student Veterinary Nurse's Name:	VN Enrolment No:
A Nonymous	1234

1. Case number-identification:

BFA 1

2. Case details:

Species: Canine *Breed:* Jack Russell Terrier
Sex: Male (Neutered) *Age:* 10yrs *Weight:* 9kg

3. History:

Sam was presented with a deep incised wound sustained to the right foreleg, whilst out on exercise with his owner.

4. Clinical evaluation of patient:

- Moderate arterial haemorrhage from deep incision to palmar aspect of right foreleg proximal to metacarpal pad, approximately 4cm in length.
- Slightly ataxic but still standing.
- Patient was observed to be shivering with cold extremities.
- Pale mucous membranes.
- Capillary refill time – 2 seconds.
- Tachypnoea/tachycardia.
- Remained alert and responsive.

5. First aid procedure carried out:

- Owner arrived unexpectedly – no veterinary surgeon on premises.
- Patient wrapped in blanket to conserve body heat.
- Owner restrained patient whilst I applied a sterile dressing (Melorin; Smith+Nephew) to the wound and a pressure bandage (1 layer of cotton wool over the whole foot, extra layer of cotton wool over wounded area, conforming bandage over whole foot and white cohesive bandage as top layer). This enclosed the whole foot, extending above the carpus.
- I contacted the veterinary surgeon.
- Whilst waiting for the veterinary surgeon to arrive I observed the patient for further deterioration and reassured the client.

6. Monitoring of the animal:

- Observed patient, monitoring vital signs (temperature, pulse and respiration – see attached notes made at time).

- Observed pressure bandage to ensure that no blood was seeping through. If it had I would have applied an additional bandage on top of the first.

7. Outcome of first aid:

- No blood soaked through bandage therefore haemorrhage stemmed successfully.
- Veterinary surgeon arrived to provide further treatment.
- Wound sutured under general anaesthetic.

8. Date(s): *to include date of incident and full timescale range, if appropriate*

26.10.01 Patient admitted at 7.55am
        Veterinary surgeon arrived at 8.15am

Student's Comments: *to include confirmation of your role in the procedures and any additional detail not given previously*

The patient was discharged later that same day. I provided initial first aid care and was pleased to see how the application of the pressure bandage helped to stop the bleeding.

The evidence in this log sheet is a true representation of my involvement in the case described, and the work undertaken in compiling the log is my own.

Student Veterinary Nurse's Signature:

Assessor's Statement:

The procedures and details associated with the basic first aid described have been carried out correctly and competently by the student.

Comments:
On liaison with the attending veterinary surgeon, Mr Small, and questioning Anna about this case, I can confirm that she acted in a competent manner in dealing with this first aid incident.

Assessor's Signature: *Date:*

Assessor's Name: *Assessor's Qualifications:*

LOG SHEET 3C: ADMINISTRATION OF MEDICATION TO ANIMALS

Student Veterinary Nurse's Name:	**VN Enrolment No:**
A Nonymous	1234

1. Case number-identification:

AD MED 1

2. Case details:

Species: Feline   *Breed:* DSH (Domestic Short Hair)

Sex: Male (Neutered)   *Age:* 7yrs   *Weight:* 5kg

3. Name of drug administered: *to include trade and generic names, and classification and drug form: e.g. antibiotic/cream, sedative/injection etc.*

Domitor 'Medetomidine' sedative/injection 1mg/ml solution

4. Date administered:

1.11.01

5. Dose given: *to include calculations*

Dose rate: Medetomidine 0.1mg/kg

Dose given (including calculation): 5kg x 0.1mg = 0.5mg required

                                             1mg per 1mg therefore needs 0.5/1.0 = 0.5ml

6. Reason for administration, basic effect of the drug and how it was administered:

- Moderate sedation to allow radiographic procedure and examination to be performed.
- Administered intramuscularly into the quadriceps femoris of the hindlimb.
- The intramuscular route was chosen because the drug would be effective within 10–20min which allowed time to prepare equipment.

7. Health and safety issues and precautions taken:

If a controlled drug, specify the recording and storage requirements and attach a copy of the register entry if applicable.

- Wear gloves when drawing up and administering medetomidine.
- Put needles into sharps container as soon as they have been used.
- Use the correct method of restraint to avoid injury to personnel or patient.
- Close all doors and windows in the ward prior to getting cat out of kennel.

8. Did you process the payment for the medication correctly?

The amount of drug used was entered onto the patient's computer record which automatically calculated the cost for this injection. The total bill was paid by the client when they collected the cat later.

Student's Comments and Signature:

The administration of this drug was carried out in a safe manner. I prepared myself, the injection and the environment prior to getting the patient out of the kennel to help minimise any complications.

The evidence in this log sheet is a true representation of my involvement in the case described, and the work undertaken in compiling the log is my own.

Student Veterinary Nurse's Signature:

Assessor's Statement:

The procedures and details associated with the administration of medication described have been observed by me and have been carried out correctly and competently.

Comments:

I observed Anna administering this sedative drug intramuscularly to Fletcher. She was well prepared, calculated the correct dose and administered the drug in a confident and competent manner.

Assessor's Signature: *Date:*

Assessor's Name: *Assessor's Qualifications:*

LOG SHEET 4A: HEALTH AND SAFETY RISK ASSESSMENT

Student Veterinary Nurse's Name:	VN Enrolment No:
A Nonymous	1234

1. Animal hospitalisation area:

Work activities carried out:
- Monitoring of inpatients... feeding, grooming, exercising.
- Treatment of inpatients (administering medication, monitoring equipment such as materials used for fluid therapy, maintenance of dressings, drains etc.).
- Cleaning of kennels and hospital environment (corridors, shelves, sinks etc.).
- Disposal of waste (clinical and non-clinical).

2. Regulations that are applicable to the work activities and work area:

- Health and Safety at Work Act (1974)
- Reporting of Incidents of Disease and Dangerous Occurrences Regulations (1995)
- Control of Substances Hazardous to Health Regulations (1999)
- Misuse of Drugs Act (1971)
- Misuse of Drugs Regulations (1985)
- Control of Pollution Act (1974) ⎫
- Collection and Disposal of Waste Regulations (1988) ⎬ Clinical Waste Regulations
- Environmental Protection Act (1990) ⎭
- Health & Safety (First Aid) Regulations (1981)

3. Significant or potential hazards:

- Bites and scratches from animals if handled incorrectly
- Needles and sharp instruments
- Cleaning and disinfection of floors and surfaces (use of chemicals and wet floors)
- Transporting/carrying animals
- Electrical equipment
- Clinical waste
- Handling drugs
- Zoonotic infectious agents (e.g. leptospirosis, toxoplasmosis, ringworm)

4. People at risk:

- Veterinary surgeons
- Veterinary nurses
- Trainee veterinary nurses
- Reception staff
- Work experience students
- Clients visiting animals

5. Existing control measures:

- Staff trained to handle animals and administer medication – restraint equipment and protection available.

- Needles/sharps disposed of in yellow plastic 'sharps' bin, not exceeding maximum full line. Once full this is sealed and collected by a licensed operator.
- Spillages are dealt with immediately. Yellow cones are used to warn people of wet floors.
- Animals are transported safely and securely (on a lead or in a basket). All staff are trained in safe lifting techniques.
- Electrical equipment (e.g. clippers) is tested annually and should only be used with dry hands. Cables should be above waist height to prevent injury.
- Clinical waste is disposed of in yellow sacks marked clinical waste. These are changed on a daily basis, sealed with biohazard tape and put in the garage until they are collected by the licensed operator.
- If a zoonotic disease is suspected, our barrier nursing protocol is followed (see Appendix 3).
- Work experience students are never left unsupervised.

6. Estimated level of risk (low/medium/high, as appropriate):

Medium, providing control measures followed.

7. Suggested long-term actions:

- All new members of staff to receive health and safety training, particularly in the areas of handling animals, safe lifting and zoonotic diseases.
- Monitor adherence to control measures to confirm they are being followed.

Student's Comments:

Health and safety within the kennel area is of prime importance and has its risks. Providing the control measures are followed, these should be kept to a minimum.

The evidence in this log sheet is a true representation of my involvement in the case described, and the work undertaken in compiling the log is my own.

Student Veterinary Nurse's Signature:

Assessor's Statement:

The student has demonstrated good Health and Safety working practices associated with this Risk Assessment Report.

Comments:
Anna is aware of the health and safety requirements of the workplace and has received training as part of her induction. On questioning she demonstrated that she has a good understanding of practice procedures (see Appendix A) and I can confirm that she works safely, taking necessary precautions when required.

Assessor's Signature: *Date:*

Assessor's Name: *Assessor's Qualifications:*

LOG SHEET 4B: HUMAN HEALTH EMERGENCY (FIRST AID)

Student Veterinary Nurse's Name:	VN Enrolment No:
A Nonymous	1234

1. Details of occurrence:

Whilst holding a dog for examination, my colleague, another student veterinary nurse, was bitten on her right hand, drawing a small amount of blood.

2. Copy of incident book entry (attached): ☐ *please tick*

If the incident was not recorded please state why.

3. First aid procedure carried out:

- The dog was removed to a kennel for temporary holding whilst first aid was administered.
- I put on protective gloves from the first aid box and cleaned my colleague's wound under cold running water.
- I applied a clean sterile swab to prevent further bleeding, applying slight pressure.
- When the bleeding stopped, I put a plaster over the wound to prevent further infection.
- I advised my colleague to check the date of her last tetanus and to keep the wound clean and dry.
- I advised her to seek medical advice if the wound did not improve.

4. Student's role:

- I removed the dog to the kennel for safety so that he could do no further harm.
- I rinsed the wound, applied a swab to stop the bleeding and then applied a plaster.
- I recorded the details in the accident book.

5. Outcome:

My colleague was confident that the incident was minor and continued to restrain the dog, that was now muzzled, for further examination and treatment.

6. Date(s):

26.10.01 at approximately 10am

Student's Comments:

I administered the first aid myself under the supervision of our head nurse, Mrs V Tall VN who holds the First Aid at Work Certificate.

The evidence in this log sheet is a true representation of my involvement in the case described, and the work undertaken in compiling the log is my own.

Student Veterinary Nurse's Signature:

Assessor's Statement:

The procedures and details associated with the incident described have been carried out competently.

Comments:

Anna is competent at dealing with the majority of first aid situations that occur in practice. She has recently attended a 1 day course arranged by St John's Ambulance to improve first aid awareness (certificate enclosed).

Please state if assessment was by simulation.

Assessor's Signature: *Date:*

Assessor's Name: *Assessor's Qualifications:*

LOG SHEET 4C: SECURITY OF THE VETERINARY PRACTICE

Student Veterinary Nurse's Name:	VN Enrolment No:
A Nonymous	1234

1. What steps are taken to prevent the misuse of drugs and other medical supplies?

Schedule 2 and other addictive drugs (see Appendix 6) are stored in a locked cabinet to which only the veterinary surgeons have the key.

All drugs are kept in dispensary to which the general public do not have access. In-use injectable drugs are kept in the consulting rooms in cupboards out of view and access by the general public.

All Schedule 2 controlled drugs received, used or discarded are recorded in the dangerous drugs register.

2. What are the relevant regulations? Briefly outline how they affect the storage, display and supply of drugs.

Misuse of Drugs Act (1971) – states that all addictive drugs should be kept under lock and key and their purchase, use and disposal recorded.

Medicines Act (1968) – states that only Prescription Only Medicines may be sold by a veterinary surgeon to a client in his/her care. It governs the licensing of human and veterinary drugs in addition to medicated animal feeds. It controls the storage, dispensing and labelling of drugs and categorises them into one of 4 categories – Prescription Only Medicines (POM), including controlled drugs (CD); Pharmacy medicines (P), Pharmacy Merchants' List (PML) and General Sales List (GSL). A description of and examples from each drug category is included in Appendix 7.

3. Give three examples of equipment (veterinary or general) which you use, and summarise how risks of misuse, damage to, and theft of this equipment are minimised.

Computers – all personnel trained in their use are given passwords. All secured to walls by security chains and marked with a security pen. Windows protected by bars to prevent theft.

Safe – Access restricted, immovable, code changes regularly, records to confirm balance, secure, out of sight location.

Syringes – Correct disposal, render unfit for re-use. Access to storage site restricted.

4. What security measures are taken to protect veterinary records and how do you ensure records remain secure?

All our records are held on computer to which only authorised staff have passwords.

Files are backed up every evening and the tape is locked in a fire-proof safe to which only senior partners have keys.

All staff are aware of the Data Protection Act (1984) and the need for client confidentiality.

5. How do you ensure the security of personal possessions (belonging to you, your colleagues and your clients)?

- Each member of staff has their own locker where personal possessions can be stored. Only they have a key (the Principal of the practice has a master key so that should a key be lost, access can be obtained). All staff are instructed not to leave valuable items lying around.
- Personal possessions of clients are labelled with the client's details and await collection. If anything is of value, it is placed in the safe to which only senior partners have a key.

6. State the security systems (e.g. building alarms, etc) which you are confident and competent to use. *(Your assessor must be able to confirm this.)*

Alarm bells	Locked gates
Secure loading/unloading	Electronic doors
Key pads	Intercom system
Money safes	Intruder prevention e.g. window bars
Cameras	Drug cabinets
Mirrors	Staff lockers
Panic buttons	

Student's Comments and Signature:

I am responsible for checking all windows and entry points to the surgery are locked and secure before leaving each day.

The evidence in this log sheet is a true representation of my involvement in the case described, and the work undertaken in compiling the log is my own.

Student Veterinary Nurse's Signature:

Assessor's Statement

The procedures relating to maintaining security of the veterinary practice have been carried out competently by the candidate.

Comments:

Anna has a clear understanding of the issues surrounding personal and other security measures, when questioned on this topic she had a good underpinning knowledge of the subject (see Appendix A).

Assessor's Signature: *Date:*

Assessor's Name: *Assessor's Qualifications:*

Example case log sheets for modules 5–10

LOG SHEET 5A: LABORATORY AND DIAGNOSTIC AIDS

Student Veterinary Nurse's Name:	VN Enrolment No:
A Nonymous	1234

1. Case number-identification:

LAB 2

2. Case details:

Species: Feline   *Breed:* DSH (Domestic Short Hair)
Sex: Male (Entire)   *Age:* 7mths   *Weight:* 3kg

3. Type of procedure and reason for test:

Cystocentesis for urinalysis due to recurrent cystitis.

4. Preparation of animal and pre-test procedures:

Temperature, pulse and respiration were checked along with capillary refill time, colour of mucous membranes and skin turgor. Food had been withdrawn for 12 hours. The bladder was palpated to ensure it wasn't too empty or full. A 5cm² area was clipped on the midline caudal abdomen and cleaned aseptically with chlorhexidine.

5. Equipment and supplies required:

Clippers, gloves, dilute chlorhexidine solution and surgical spirit. Sterile 10ml syringe + 23 gauge x 12 needle. Urine collection pots: boric acid/plain, urine reagent, dipsticks, pipettes, centrifuge + tubes, microscope slides, coverslip, mounting needle.

6. Preparation of equipment:

Urinary dipsticks were checked to ensure they had not been damaged or contaminated in any way and that they were within the expiry date. The chlorhexidine solution was made fresh with warm H_2O. The clippers were lubricated and the blade checked for broken teeth. The centrifuge was switched on ready for use.

7. Collection of sample:

I restrained the patient in left and lateral recumbency, with hind legs extended caudally. The veterinary surgeon manually immobilised the bladder through the abdominal wall. He inserted the needle through the abdominal wall into the bladder and drew urine into the syringe. Once the needle was removed I applied digital pressure at the injection site.

8. Preparation of sample for testing/storage and preservation, prior to despatch:

The urine was equally divided into a plain universal container and boric acid container and the tests were immediately carried out.

9. Procedure(s) for test OR packaging and postage:
  method of despatch see guidance notes

A drop of urine was placed on each reagent strip on the urinary dipstick and read against the colour chart at the appropriate times. Urine was transferred to 3/4 fill two centrifuge tubes and the samples were spun for 4min @ 400rpm using a microhaematocrit centrifuge. The supernatant fluid was removed using a sterile pipette and the sediment was then transferred onto a microscope slide and a coverslip applied. It was then examined under a microscope.

10. Results of test:

pH 7.0   Ketones negative   Specific gravity 1.008
Blood +++   Glucose negative   Microscopy: triple phosphate crystals seen
Protein ++   Urobilinogen negative

11. Normal ranges:

pH 6–7   Specific gravity 1.020–1.040
A little protein + urobilinogen can be normal, everything else should appear negative.

12. Examples of conditions which may give rise to abnormal ranges:

1. Blood: cystitis, neoplasia, nephritis
2. Specific gravity (decrease): pyometra, diabetes insipidus, increased H_2O intake
3. Protein: haematuria, pyuria, cystitis
4. Struvite/triple phosphate crystals: staphylococcal infections, alkaline urine

13. Possible reasons for inaccurate results:

Reading results at the wrong time; dipsticks out of date; alkaline urine can affect protein result; prolonged storage.

14. Date(s) sample collected and test carried out:

5.6.02 – sample collected. Test conducted immediately.

Student's Comments and Signature:

Urine must be tested immediately when at all possible, or preserved. Cystocentesis is the preferred method for obtaining urine for analysis as, if carried out correctly, it is the most sterile method.

The evidence in this log sheet is a true representation of my involvement in the case described, and the work undertaken in compiling the log is my own.

Student Veterinary Nurse's Signature:

Assessor's Statement:

The nursing procedures and monitoring of the medical case described have been observed by me and have been carried out correctly and competently.

Comments:
Anna routinely performs urinalysis at the request of the veterinary surgeon. She is competent in relation to unit 8 of the occupational standards with regard to this procedure.

Assessor's Signature: *Date:*

Assessor's Name: *Assessor's Qualifications:*

LOG SHEET 5B: MAINTAINING LABORATORY EQUIPMENT

Student Veterinary Nurse's Name:	VN Enrolment No:
A Nonymous	1234

1. Give details of the equipment used:

Partfocal binocular microscope.

2. State the make of equipment used in your practice:

SWIFT M4000-D

3. Describe the procedure for the cleaning, maintenance and sterilisation, if appropriate, of this equipment:

Monthly cleaning regime:

1. Remove each eyepiece and clean with cotton bud and industrial methylated spirit to remove grease. Polish with lens cloth and replace.

2. Remove each objective lens and treat as above. Methylated spirit is used sparingly as it can soften the lens mounting over time.

3. Clean stage using mild detergent (Decon 90), rinse and dry.

4. Clean substage condenser with lens cloth and glass above light source.

5. Gently wipe the remainder of the microscope with a damp cloth.

6. All moving parts are oiled e.g. rack.

Routine maintenance: The stage is cleaned after each use. The oil immersion lens is cleaned after each use. The microscope is placed in a box if not in use to avoid dust/debris accumulation.

4. State three faults which may occur with this equipment:

1. Failure of light source – lightbulb would need replacing.

2. Damage/chipping of lenses during cleaning – may need to replace lens.

3. Seizure of moving parts – may need to be sent to manufacturer for service/repair.

5. Give details of the action that should be taken in the event of a malfunction:

If malfunction occurs I would try to identify the reasons for the malfunction. If it is a light source failure, the fuse in the plug should be replaced and the bulb if necessary.

If the stage is seized, lubrication may be required.

If I was unable to rectify the problem I would report the malfunction to the Principal and arrange for it to be serviced/repaired by the manufacturer.

Student's Comments and Signature:

As a trainee it is my responsibility to regularly clean the microscope on a monthly basis and ensure others clean it after use. Regular maintenance is important as it prolongs the life of the equipment in practice.

The evidence in this log sheet is a true representation of my involvement in the case described, and the work undertaken in compiling the log is my own.

Student Veterinary Nurse's Signature:

Assessor's Statement:

The procedures and details associated described have been observed by me and have been carried out correctly and competently.

Comments:

Anna has been given the responsibility of maintaining lab equipment since covering the underpinning knowledge at college. She is now confident in cleaning all the parts of the microscope and performs this to a high standard, providing evidence towards unit 8.1 and 14.2 of the occupational standard.

Assessor's Signature: *Date:*

Assessor's Name: *Assessor's Qualifications:*

LOG SHEET 6A: MEDICAL NURSING

Student Veterinary Nurse's Name:	VN Enrolment No:
A Nonymous	1234

1. Case number-identification:

14997

2. Case details:

Species: Canine   *Breed:* West Highland White Terrier
Sex: Male (Neutered)   *Age:* 8yrs   *Weight:* 7.4kg

3. Major presenting problem and history:

No significant clinical history until seven days ago when he started to vomit. Has been vomiting ever since, he is now unable to keep any food or water down and is dehydrated. The dog escaped and went missing for a few hours about a week ago.

4. Principal clinical findings:

On clinical examination the dog was dehydrated. He had very dry mucous membranes and his skin was starting to tent. He had a temperature of 39.5°C and was generally very depressed and lethargic. No other abnormalities were detected on physical examination.

5. Diagnostic procedures and tests:

a State procedures and test(s) carried out in order to assist in the diagnosis of the condition.

b Describe your involvement with these procedures.

The dog was admitted to carry out further investigations.

First a blood sample was obtained from the dog's right jugular vein. I assisted by holding the patient whilst the vet took the sample. The blood was then analysed in our in-house laboratory. I assisted in running a biochemistry and haematology assay on the sample (see laboratory log sheets 5A). As soon as results were ready I took them to the vet for interpretation. There was nothing of significance apart from a raised packed cell volume (PCV), which would be expected, as the dog was dehydrated.

The next investigation was to perform radiography (see radiography log sheet 7A). The radiographs revealed that the dog had an oesophageal foreign body, which looked like a bone from the radiographs.

6. Comment on clinical findings, test results and veterinary surgeon's diagnosis:

Initial clinical finding of dehydration was likely to be due to the fact that the dog was continually vomiting and unable to keep any fluids or food down.

The blood tests were useful as they ruled out the possibility of any systemic disease that may have been causing the dog to vomit. The radiographs were very useful as they confirmed a diagnosis.

The veterinary surgeon's diagnosis was an oesophageal foreign body.

7. Medical treatment and nursing: *to include medication and other treatments prescribed; dietary management; monitoring of progress and response to treatments; *fluid therapy *(details can be expanded in log sheet 6b)*

The dog was hospitalised for four days post removal of the foreign body. I was responsible for the nursing care of the dog which included:

Administering prescribed medication which was
- Sucralfate (Antepsin) 1g tablet was given three times daily by mouth.
- Cimetidine (Tagamet) 100mg was given three times daily by mouth.
- Amoxycillin/clavulanate (Synulox) 125mg was given twice daily by mouth.

The dog received fluid therapy for the first three days post removal of foreign body (see log sheet 6b).

Due to receiving fluid therapy the dog had an intravenous catheter in place. I checked this three times daily for patency by flushing with a small amount of heparinised saline. I also checked for any signs of dislodgement, redness or swelling that would have indicated an infection. The catheter was kept bandaged at all times to prevent patient interference.

For the first two days the dog was on nil per os, this was to allow the oesophagus time to recover as it may have been damaged by the foreign body and removal of it. Once feeding commenced I offered the dog Hills a/d that was soft and easy to swallow and also rich in calories and easily digestible postoperatively. The dog was fed approximately 50g six times daily.

The dog was observed closely at all times for any signs of vomiting. Should the dog start to vomit the vet was to be informed immediately. Fortunately this did not occur.

The dog was taken to a grass area four times a day to allow him to urinate and defaecate.

8. Case summary and evaluation: *e.g. the outcome, your role in case, information given to clients*

The dog made a good recovery and was discharged five days after removal of the foreign body. He was to continue the medication that he received whilst hospitalised for a further four days and was to be re-examined one week after discharge.

When the dog was discharged the vet explained to the owner what tests and procedures the dog had undergone whilst hospitalised and showed the bone. I then had to explain how to administer the medication and go through the doses. I also explained that he should continue on Hills a/d until he came back for his re-exam.

My role in this case was to assist the vet with the initial examination and blood tests. I also assisted while the dog was under general anaesthesia. I nursed the dog for the time whilst he was hospitalised.

9. Date(s): *to include full timescale range, if appropriate*

Admitted 03.09.01
Discharged 08.09.01

Student's Comments and Signature:

This was a very interesting case to nurse and I learnt a lot about nursing patients after foreign body removal.

The evidence in this log sheet is a true representation of my involvement in the case described, and the work undertaken in compiling the log is my own.

Student Veterinary Nurse's signature:

Assessor's Statement:

The nursing procedures and monitoring of the medical case described have been observed by me and have been carried out correctly and competently.

Comments:
Anna demonstrated good nursing practise during the care of this case and has a good underpinning knowledge demonstrated by questioning (see Appendix A).

Assessor's Signature: *Date:*

Assessor's Name: *Assessor's Qualifications:*

LOG SHEET 6B: FLUID MANAGEMENT

Student Veterinary Nurse's Name:	VN Enrolment No:
A Nonymous	1234

1. Case number-identification:

14997

2. Case details:

Species: Canine   *Breed:* West Highland White Terrier

Sex: Male (Neutered)   *Age:* 8yrs   *Weight:* 7.4kg

3. Reason for administering fluid:

Dehydrated due to vomiting for five days, this was due to an oesophageal foreign body, which was removed via endoscopy.

4. Type of fluid selected: *according to veterinary surgeon's instructions*

0.9% sodium chloride (NaCl) solution

5. Reason for choice of fluid and route of administration:

The veterinary surgeon chose 0.9% NaCl solution as it is useful for replacing water and electrolyte losses in vomiting patients. It is a crystalloid solution. I administered the fluid by the intravenous route, under instruction of the veterinary surgeon.

6. Equipment and supplies: *state what was selected and how it was prepared in order to administer the fluids*

I prepared the following equipment for use:

A 500ml bag of 0.9% NaCl, an administration (giving) set, a 20g intravenous catheter, elastoplast tape, cotton wool, scrub solution and clippers.

I connected the administration set to the bag of fluids in a sterile manner and ran the fluid through the administration set to remove any air.

The intravenous catheter was placed in the patient's left cephalic vein by the veterinary surgeon after it had been clipped and scrubbed. This was secured in place using elastoplast tape.

7. Fluid therapy plan:

a. Estimated total fluid deficit.

b. Rate of administration (include ml per hour and drip rate).

Show how volume (a) and rates (b) were calculated.

Replacement: inevitable losses (20ml/kg/day) 20 x 7.4 x 5 = 740ml

Vomiting for 5 days (4ml/kg/vomit) 4 x 7.4 x 15 = 444ml

Urinary water loss (20ml/kg/day) 20 x 7.4 x 2 = 296ml

Total water deficit = 1480ml

1/3rd of this is ECF = 493ml

Replacement required (plasma deficit) = 123ml

Maintenance (50ml/kg/day) 50 x 7.4 x 1 = 370ml

Total volume required = 493ml

Using a standard administration set (20 drops/ml) the fluid rate is:

$\dfrac{493}{24}$ = 20.5ml per hour

$\dfrac{20.5}{60}$ = 0.34ml per min

20 x 0.34 = 6.8 drops per min

8. Summary of fluid therapy plan: *any revisions to the initial plan*

After two days of fluid therapy the dog was recovering well. The rate of infusion was reduced to 400ml a day as the dog was urinating well. On day three the dog was offered food which he readily took. Once he was eating well and not vomiting the fluids were gradually weaned down to be removed on day four.

9. Monitoring of the animal:

a Monitoring of administration, urine output, vital signs etc. and animal's progress.

b A recording chart/record used by you to monitor this animal must be attached.

I monitored the dog throughout his hospitalisation. I marked the fluid bag with pen as to how much he should receive each day. I checked the drip regularly to ensure that it was still dripping and the catheter was checked three times daily to ensure patency and that there were no signs of infection.

The dog initially produced very little urine as he was dehydrated, but as his fluid deficit was corrected he started to urinate regularly. Over time the dog became brighter and more alert. The dog improved well once he was rehydrated and eating.

10. Date(s): *to include full timescale range, if appropriate*

Admitted 03.09.01

Discharged 08.09.01

Student's Comments and Signature:

The patient did not interfere with his intravenous catheter, but if he had I could have placed an Elizabethan collar to prevent him from chewing or pulling it out.

The evidence in this log sheet is a true representation of my involvement in the case described, and the work undertaken in compiling the log is my own.

Student Veterinary Nurse's Signature:

Assessor's Statement:

The procedures and details associated with the fluid management described have been observed by me and have been carried out correctly and competently.

Comments:
Anna has shown much improvement in calculating drip rates since covering the underpinning knowledge at college. She can now do this without any help apart from confirmation that her calculation is correct prior to administering fluids.

Assessor's Signature: *Date:*

Assessor's Name: .   *Assessor's Qualifications:*

LOG SHEET 7A: RADIOGRAPHY

Student Veterinary Nurse's Name: A Nonymous	VN Enrolment No: 1234

1. Case number-identification:

RAD 7a 1

2. Case details:

Species: Canine *Breed:* Labrador Retriever
Sex: F(Neutered) *Age:* 8yrs *Weight:* 26kg

3. Area to be radiographed and reason:

Sudden lameness on L hind – suspect cruciate ligament rupture – radiograph L stifle

4. Patient preparation:
to include means of restraint e.g. manual, chemical (state medication used)

General anaesthesia
Pre-med – 0.4 Acp/0.4ml Buprenorphine
Induction agent – Rapinovet 16ml
Maintained on Isoflo/oxygen via a circle circuit

5. Recording equipment:

Screen Type: Rare Earth Film Type: Screen Film Grid: Focussed

6. Exposure factors:

FFD: 75cm kV: 70 mAs: 0.12mAs

7. View e.g. ventro dorsal:

Lateral stifle

8. Positioning of animal: *to include positioning aids used*

The patient was laid in left lateral recumbancy in a radiolucent trough – her R hind limb was secured out of the tray using a tie and a sand bag was used to prevent rotation of the stifle.

9. Centring details: *state anatomical landmarks*

I centred on the stifle joint space.

10. Collimation of primary beam: *state anatomical landmarks*

I collimated to include the distal third of the femur and the proximal third of the tibia/fibula.

I collimated to include the skin surfaces.

11. Appraisal of radiographical quality:
   to include action taken in respect of any faults identified

The radiograph was of diagnostic quality, although my collimation could have been much tighter. The exposure was fine and due to a well-maintained automatic processor. The radiograph had no processing faults.

12. Veterinary surgeon's diagnosis:

No ruptured cruciate ligament was seen, or anything else on the radiograph.

Diagnosis – severe soft tissue damage of the area.

13. Date radiograph taken:

19.12.01

Student's Comments and Signature:

I never really enjoyed radiography, but doing these cases means that I have to practice positioning etc. I am becoming more confident in this area.

The evidence in this log sheet is a true representation of my involvement in the case described, and the work undertaken in compiling the log is my own.

Student Veterinary Nurse's Signature:

Assessor's Statement:

The procedures and details associated with the radiographic procedure described have been observed by me and have been carried out correctly and competently.

Comments:
Anna is learning quickly how important it is to position well for radiography; she is improving all the time with practice. She explained the pre-med that was used as I felt this was unclear in the case log sheet presented.

Assessor's Signature: *Date:*

Assessor's Name: *Assessor's Qualifications:*

LOG SHEET 7B: HEALTH & SAFETY RISK ASSESSMENT
FOR RADIOGRAPHY

Student Veterinary Nurse's Name:	VN Enrolment No:
A Nonymous	1234

1. Radiographic procedures undertaken:

Work activities (shown on other Risk Assess logs).

Exposure of patients/staff to ionising radiation.

Frequency: Daily

2. Regulations that are applicable to the work activity and work area:

- Ionising Radiations Regulations (1999)
- Practice Local Rules

3. Significant hazards:

- Primary beam
- Scattered radiation
- Tube head

4. People at risk:

- Staff as listed in the Local Rules
- Patients

5. Existing control measures:

- Lead lined table/X-ray cassettes
- 2m controlled area around the 1° beam
- All patients are anaesthetised
- Dosemeters are worn and checked monthly
- Grids are used on areas over 10cm thick

6. Estimated level of risk (low/medium/high, as appropriate):

Low

7. Suggested long-term actions:

To stick with the existing control measures as the dosemeter readings are all 0–0.

The Local Rules should be updated regularly – e.g. new staff should be added.

All new staff should be trained in the correct procedures.

Student's Comments and Signature:

Health and safety can easily be overlooked in practice. I am pleased that my practice takes radiation H&S so seriously.

The evidence in this log sheet is a true representation of my involvement in the case described, and the work undertaken in compiling the log is my own.

Student Veterinary Nurse's signature:

Assessor's Statement:

The student has completed the work associated with this Risk Assessment Report, and has a thorough understanding of the knowledge and information provided.

Comments:

Anna has carried out the risk assessment well. She could have made more comment about reducing scattered radiation, although I confirmed her understanding of this with oral questions (see Appendix A).

Assessor's Signature: *Date:*

Assessor's Name: *Assessor's Qualifications:*

LOG SHEET 8A: MAINTAINING ASEPSIS

Student Veterinary Nurse's Name:	VN Enrolment No:
A Nonymous	1234

1. Procedures to be carried out in order to maintain asepsis and sterility in theatre:

a. Daily:

- At the start of each day all surfaces, furniture and equipment are damp dusted with the correct dilution of disinfectant.
- At the end of each operation the operating table is cleaned of any debris and wiped clean with disinfectant.
- Between operating the floor is cleaned of any clinical waste e.g. blood, faeces or urine.
- Bins are emptied as and when necessary or at the end of each operating day.
- At the end of each operating day the theatre is vacuumed to remove any hair and debris. The floor is washed with Trigene at a dilution of 1:50.
- Unnecessary personnel are not permitted in theatre. Theatre is an end room and not a thoroughfare to another part of the practice. Movement is kept to a minimum.
- Cloths and mop heads are washed daily.
- Surgical instruments are sterilised ready for the next operation.

b. Weekly:

All the daily procedures are carried out plus:
- A more thorough cleaning procedure is carried out: walls are cleaned with Trigene (1:50 dilution) from floor to ceiling.
- Floors are scrubbed. Trigene is active against a wide range of bacteria including Pseudomonas spp.
- All cleaning apparatus is exclusive to the theatre.
- All equipment is checked daily and at the end of each week to ensure availability and if it's in working order.
- Instruments are checked daily and weekly for damage.

c. Monthly:

All daily and weekly procedures are carried out plus:
- All surgically bagged instruments are checked for dates, tears and holes in the bag. Instruments sterilised over 3 months previously or in bags that contain holes/tears are removed and sterilised.

2. Protocol to be adopted in theatre for maintaining asepsis:

a. Preoperatively:

- Surgical personnel wear theatre suits, hats and masks.

- Surgeons and surgical assistants scrub and wear sterile gowns and gloves prior to operating.
- Patients are clipped and the initial skin preparation is performed outside of theatre in the preparation room.
- All equipment needed is sterilised (if required).
- Clean operations are performed first; those surgeries that include aural, oral or anal entry are performed last.
- A sterile surgical kit is used for each operation.

b. During operations:

- Only those members of the surgical team who are scrubbed touch the sterile instruments and equipment.
- Theatre temperature is maintained at an ambient temperature to reduce the risk of producing conditions that will encourage bacterial growth.
- Non-sterile equipment is kept away from the surgical site and team to prevent a break in asepsis.
- All contaminated instruments are removed or placed away from the sterile surgical kit.
- Clinical waste is disposed of correctly.

c. Postoperatively:

- An effective sterilisation protocol is used.
- Effective cleaning procedures are used.
- Instruments are cleaned and sterilised for the next procedure.

Student's Comments and Signature:

This is an area of work with which I am routinely involved when assisting our surgical nurse. It is important to follow the correct procedures to in order that asepsis of the theatre is maintained.

The evidence in this log sheet is a true representation of my involvement in the case described, and the work undertaken in compiling the log is my own.

Student Veterinary Nurse's Signature:

Assessor's Statement:

The student nurse has demonstrated that s/he is able to maintain an aseptic environment in relation to surgical procedures.

Comments:
Anna routinely performs all the procedures associated with maintaining asepsis in theatre and has a good appreciation of the reasons for such procedures.

Assessor's Signature: *Date:*

Assessor's Name: *Assessor's Qualifications:*

LOG SHEET 8Bi: STERILISATION USING AN AUTOCLAVE

Student Veterinary Nurse's Name:	VN Enrolment No:
A Nonymous	1234

1. Describe the type of autoclave used at your practice:

Model: Andromeda
Type: Vacuum autoclave

2. List the equipment and supplies that may be sterilised by autoclave:

- Swabs
- Metal instruments
- Metal drums
- Gowns
- Some plastics
- Drapes
- Most rubber items

3. State how the items are packaged for sterilisation:

Stainless steel instruments – on stainless steel trays (open kits) or in 'peel and seal' bags.

Browne TST chemical indicator strip – used for open kits to ensure adequate sterilisation.

Peel and seal bags have their own chemical indicator.

Swabs and drapes – sterilised in metal drum.

4. For two different items that have differing sterilisation or packaging requirements, describe the procedure:

Name of item: 2 x backhaus towel clips
Packaging used: 'peel and seal' bag

Procedure:
- Instruments washed prior to sterilisation in warm water to remove debris and placed in an ultrasonic cleaner containing 1% solution of Medigene (a proteolytic enzyme cleaner) for 3min.
- Instruments rinsed with clean water and dried thoroughly.
- Towel clips placed in 'peel and seal' bag (with ratchets open).
- Bag placed on metal tray in autoclave.
- Door firmly closed and setting selected.

Working pressure: 30psi   Temperature: 134°C   Sterilising time: 3.5min

Name of item: Bitch spay kit (see surgical Appendix 2)
Packaging used: Stainless steel tray

Procedure:
- Instruments cleaned and dried as above.
- Instrument placed on metal tray (ratchets open).
- Tray placed on a rack (holding 4 kits) in autoclave. TST strip included.

- Door closed firmly and cycle set.

Working pressure: 30psi   Temperature: 134°C   Sterilising time: 3.5min

5. Give examples of why sterilisation may be inefficient:

- Dirty instruments – all instruments should be free from grease and protein material to allow steam to penetrate.
- Autoclave too full therefore steam unable to penetrate.
- Incorrect packaging of instruments.
- Incorrect cycle selected.
- Machine not functioning correctly (pressure and temperature not achieved).

6. How do you monitor the effectiveness of the sterilisation process?

- TST strips
- 'Peel and seal' bags have chemical indicator

7. State two advantages and two disadvantages of sterilisation using an autoclave:

Advantages:

- Fast
- Easy to operate

Disadvantages:

- Equipment is very hot when removed from autoclave
- Expensive to purchase

Student's Comments and Signature:

I use the autoclave on a daily basis and find it very easy and efficient to use.

The evidence in this log sheet is a true representation of my involvement in the case described, and the work undertaken in compiling the log is my own.

Student Veterinary Nurse's Signature:

Assessor's Statement:

The student nurse has demonstrated that s/he is competent to carry out the sterilisation procedures described.

Comments:
Anna uses this piece of equipment on a daily basis and is competent in its use and maintenance. When questioned she had a good underpinning knowledge of the principles involved in sterilisation of equipment (see Appendix A).

Assessor's Signature: *Date:*

Assessor's Name: *Assessor's Qualifications:*

LOG SHEET 8Bii: STERILISATION
(OTHER THAN BY USING AN AUTOCLAVE)

Student Veterinary Nurse's Name:	VN Enrolment No:
A Nonymous	1234

1. State the method of sterilisation:

Cold chemical sterilisation using Hibitane (chlorhexidine gluconate 4%).

100ml Hibitane mixed with 150ml water made up to 1L with alcohol.

Instruments are soaked for 2mins.

2. Describe the equipment used to carry out this sterilisation:
to include details of model and type if appropriate

Plastic container for solution and instrument and measuring jug to measure out solutions.

Model: Not appropriate
Type: Not appropriate

3. Describe any other supplies used to carry out this sterilisation:

None

4. State what articles are sterilised by this method:

Instruments, tubing and plastic objects.

5. Describe the procedure for sterilisation using this equipment:
to include working pressure, temperature and sterilising times (if appropriate)

Sterilising time – soak equipment for 2mins.

6. State any advantages and disadvantages, and discuss the limitations, if any, of this method of sterilisation:

Advantages:
- Quick and easy method
- Can be used in the field
- Cheap
- Limited supplies needed

Disadvantages:
- No guarantee of sterility
- No way of checking sterility
- Can be messy

Student's Comments and Signature:

Sometimes we have to use this method to sterilise instruments although it is not a way that should be practised regularly.

The evidence in this log sheet is a true representation of my own practical work and associated knowledge.

Student Veterinary Nurse's Signature:

Assessor's Statement:

The student nurse has demonstrated that s/he is competent to carry out the sterilisation procedures described.

Comments:
This is not a method used routinely, although Anna is aware of the circumstances when it may be required.

Assessor's Signature: *Date:*

Assessor's Name: *Assessor's Qualifications:*

LOG SHEET 8C: SURGICAL NURSING – GENERAL

Student Veterinary Nurse's Name: A Nonymous	VN Enrolment No: 1234

1. Case number-identification:

SNG 1

2. Case details:

Species: Canine   *Breed:* Crossbreed
Sex: Male (Entire)   *Age:* 12yrs   *Weight:* 20kg

3. Surgical procedure:

Laryngeal tie back (left sided)

4. Preparation of instruments, surgical equipment and materials:

- Sterile bitch spay kit (see surgical Appendix 2) removed in aseptic manner from autoclave following sterilisation (134°C, 30psi for 6min). Brownes TST strip used to confirm correct sterilisation achieved.
- Other instruments, swabs and drapes placed in 'seal and peel' bags for sterilisation as above. Bags have indicator strips to ensure correct sterilisation achieved.
- Selection of suture material included:
  Ethilon – size 2 metric (polyamide filament, non-absorbable)
  Prolene – size 3 metric (polypropylene monofilament)
  Saffil – size 2 metric (polyglycolic acid, coated, braided, absorbable surgical suture)
  These were all pre-packed and sterilised by the manufacturer.
- Sterile no. 10 and no. 11 scalpel blades were also used by the veterinary surgeon.

Other equipment used included:
- 18 gauge intravenous catheter.
- Spiral giving set.
- 1L Hartmann's intravenous fluid (compound sodium lactate).
- Pulse oxymeter – to monitor blood oxygen levels and heart rate throughout procedure.
- Oesophageal stethoscope – to monitor heart rate and to indicate if the oesophagus is entered during surgery.
- Clip-on light source.
- Hand-held light source.

5. Preparation of the animal for surgery:

Pre-medication 2 hours prior to surgery:

- ACP (acepromazine maleate, sedative) 0.5ml

- Buprenorphine (analgesic) 0.6ml
- Synulox (amoxycillin/clavulanate, broad spectrum antibiotic) 1ml
- Dexadreson (corticosteriod/anti-inflamatory) 2ml

Induction of anaesthesia:
- 10ml Propofol (rapinovet – dose rate 0.5ml/kg bodyweight) via intravenous injection
- Dog intubated with size 9 endotracheal tube (cuffed)

Maintenance of anaesthesia:
- 2% isoflurane and 1L oxygen
- Initially given 4L oxygen, reduced to 1L after 10min
- Delivered via Humphrey's ADE re-breathing circuit

Preparation of the surgical site:
- Site clipped with oster A5 clippers.
- Area cleaned with Hibiscrub (chlorhexadine) (diluted 1:20 with water).
- Dog moved into operating theatre and site cleaned again with same dilution of Hibiscrub (chlorhexadine). Area dried and sprayed with Vetasept (chlorhexadine gluconate solution in 70% industrial methylated spirit).

A pulse oxymeter was attached to the tongue and oesophageal stethoscope inserted.

Dog positioned in right lateral recumbancy, forelimbs drawn caudally and held with a tie. The head and neck were extended forward and secured in position using micropore tape. The veterinary surgeon draped the patient with sterile drapes.

6. Assisting during the surgical procedure:

Fluid therapy:
- Administered via intravenous catheter (18 gauge) and spiral giving set.
- Hartmann's administered at 'surgical rate' of 10ml/kg bodyweight/hr, i.e. 200ml/hr.

Anaesthesia:
- I was responsible for maintaining a good level of anaesthesia throughout surgery.
- Heart rate monitored via the oesophageal stethoscope and pulse oxymeter.
- Oxygen saturation monitored via pulse oxymeter.
- Temperature, femoral pulse and repiratory rate were also monitored.

The veterinary surgeon had to inspect the larynx during the procedure and consequently the patient had to be extubated. I prepared 5ml of propofol (dose 5ml/kg bodyweight) for emergency use should the patient show signs of waking from anaesthesia. This was not used. The animal was intubated again by a qualified VN under instruction of the veterinary surgeon.

7. Recovery from surgery: *to include postoperative care*

I remained with the dog following surgery until it was fully conscious. He was placed in a kennel next to an oxygen point in case of respiratory distress. The kennel was lined with newspaper with vetbed for bedding. The dog was covered with bubble wrap to retain heat and prevent hypothermia.

I medicated the dog (every 6hr for 12hr post surgery) with 0.6ml Buprenorphine via intramuscular injection, under the supervision of my assessor. The following day I administered a subcutaneous injection of Synulox with tablets (250mg) being dispensed when the dog went home (1 tablet twice daily).

The dog was offered food approximately 4 hours postoperatively. He was given small amounts of Hills I/D every 2 hours that was gradually increased to 2 tins every 24 hours.

Due to the nature of the surgical site and surgery a normal collar and lead was not appropriate when exercised so a harness was used.

8. Date(s): *to include full timescale range if appropriate*

9.10.01 – 10.10.01

Student's Comments and Signature:

I was responsible for preparing the instruments, equipment and materials for this case in addition to preparing the surgical site and positioning the animal for surgery. I monitored the anaesthesia during surgery along with the fluid administered. I also observed the animal during its recovery and was solely responsible for its postoperative care until discharged (except during the night, when the night nurse was responsible).

The evidence in this log sheet is a true representation of my involvement in the case described, and the work undertaken in compiling the log is my own.

Student Veterinary Nurse's Signature:

Assessor's Statement:

The procedures and details associated with the surgical nursing described have been observed by me and have been carried out correctly and competently.

Comments:
Anna demonstrated competence in the surgical nursing of this case. Her underpinning knowledge has been confirmed with questions (see Appendix A) and I can confirm that she has a good understanding of this aspect of surgical nursing.

We have discussed the need to express drug doses in mg/ml rather than quantity administered for future case logs to avoid potential confusion.

Assessor's Signature: *Date:*

Assessor's Name: *Assessor's Qualifications:*

LOG SHEET 8D: MAINTAINING EQUIPMENT

Student Veterinary Nurse's Name:	VN Enrolment No:
A Nonymous	1234

1. Give details of the equipment used: *include name and make of equipment*

Clippers: Oster A5
Blades: No. 40

2. Describe the procedure for preparing it for use:

- Check the clipper body for any damage.
- Check the electrical lead and plug for damage or fraying of the lead.
- Remove the blades, if attached to the clippers, and check that no teeth are broken and all screws are tight. Clean blades if necessary.
- Plug the clippers in and turn on. Check the clippers look and sound in working order.

They are now ready for use.

3. Describe the procedure for the cleaning and maintenance of this equipment:

- Unplug the clippers from the mains.
- Remove the blades from the clippers.
- Clean and disinfect the clipper blades.
- Brush any hair away from the moving parts of the clippers and spray with clipper oil.
- Place the clipper blades back onto the clippers, then turn on the clippers and snap the blades back into position. Spray the moving blades with clipper oil.

They are now ready for use.

4. Describe the procedure for sterilisation of the equipment (if appropriate):

The only part of the clippers that you can sterilise is the clipper blades. This would be done by placing the blades in a bag or container and sterilising in an autoclave or hot air oven. Chemical sterilisation could also be performed.

5. State three faults that may occur with this equipment:

1. Broken teeth – these clipper blades should be disposed of. Using these blades could bruise or cut the skin of the patient.
2. Electrical or fuse failure.
3. Loose wires within the body of the clippers.

6. Give details of the action that should be taken in the event of malfunction:

In the event of a malfunction of the clippers I would unplug them and label them "DO NOT USE". I would then remove the clippers and put them in a safe place and inform our head nurse. The clippers would be sent away to the manufacturers for repair.

Student's Comments and Signature:

This case taught me it is essential to keep equipment available and working in a busy veterinary practice. Therefore, it is essential that everyone knows what to do if a malfunction occurs.

The evidence in this log sheet is a true representation of my involvement in the case described, and the work undertaken in compiling the log is my own.

Student Veterinary Nurse's Signature:

Assessor's Statement:

The equipment described is as used at this training centre.

The student nurse is competent to:

- *prepare it for use,*
- *clean, sterilise and store it (as appropriate), and*
- *identify and report malfunction (as appropriate).*

Comments:
Clippers receive a great deal of wear and tear in the practice. Anna has the responsibility to ensure that they are regularly maintained, which she performs competently on a routine basis.

Assessor's Signature: *Date:*

Assessor's Name: *Assessor's Qualifications:*

LOG SHEET 9A: ANAESTHESIA

Student Veterinary Nurse's Name:	VN Enrolment No:
A Nonymous	1234

1. Case number-identification:

ANAES 1

2. Case details:

Species: Canine *Breed:* Border Collie
Sex: Bitch *Age:* 10yrs 5mths *Weight:* 24.6kg

3. Description of animal:
including general health status and any pre-existing conditions

The patient is an insulin-dependent diabetic diagnosed three months ago. She is stable except during oestrus. She is in good body condition and has a good coat. She is a little nervous and can kennel guard.

4. Reason for anaesthesia/procedure:

To perform an ovario-hysterectomy to help in regulation of the diabetes.

5. Preparation of the anaesthetic equipment and supplies:
e.g. anaesthetic machine, circuit, drugs, monitoring equipment, gas scavenging etc.

It was my responsibility to carry out the following tasks:

- Check anaesthetic machine including level of anaesthetic gases, oxygen and nitrous oxide.
- Select an anaesthetic circuit and attach to machine – in this case I selected a circle and confirmed that this was acceptable with the veterinary surgeon.
- I calculated the amount of induction agent (Rapinovet: Propofol) to be administered (under veterinary supervision) (see Appendix 1).
- Lay out a range of endotracheal tubes and a laryngoscope.
- Check monitoring equipment (pulse-oximeter and oesophageal stethoscope).
- Attach the scavenging system (passive).

6. Preoperative preparation of the animal:

I was responsible for ensuring that the following preparation occurred preoperatively:

- I confirmed with the owner that the patient had been starved preoperatively for 12 hours and that she had been given half her normal dose of insulin on the morning of the operation. I also confirmed that she had not been given her breakfast on the morning of the operation.

- On admittance, under supervision of our surgical nurse, I placed an over-the-needle catheter in the right cephalic vein and a took a blood sample for a glucose test. This was recorded on her anaesthetic record chart.
- Under direction of the veterinary surgeon I premedicated the patient with 0.3mg Acepromazine and 50mg Pethidine 30min prior to induction. Carprophen was also given at this time (98mg). After the premedication the patient was more relaxed and calm in her kennel.

7. Student's comments: *to include induction and maintenance of anaesthesia, and your role during the procedure. Give reasons for the veterinary surgeon's choice of anaesthetic agents and circuits and comment on any unusual features of this case.*

- The patient was induced with 98mg propofol given intravenously and maintained on 1.5% isoflurane and 2L oxygen.
- A circle circuit was used because the patient was over 20kg and a low flow rate of oxygen can be used. Therefore for bigger dogs this reduces the cost of anaesthesia.
- Propofol was used as an induction agent because it is rapidly metabolised and does not linger in the system. Therefore the animal should recover from anaesthesia quicker than when using some other agents. Isoflurane was also used for this reason. The patient needed to recover rapidly from the anaesthetic because she needed to be fed her breakfast to prevent a hypoglycaemic (low blood glucose) attack from occurring.
- I monitored the anaesthetic and took blood glucose samples every 15min until the patient was fully recovered. After she had eaten they were taken every hour. It is very important to monitor glucose levels in diabetic dogs especially under anaesthesia when it would be difficult to notice the signs of a hypoglycaemic attack. Low blood glucose levels for a lengthy period can cause brain damage.

8. Student's comments: *to include recovery*

- The patient's recovery was rapid and uneventful.
- I gave her her normal amount of breakfast (brought in by her owners) 45min postoperatively.
- Her blood glucose began to increase significantly during the afternoon and she was given a small dose of soluble insulin to counteract this prior to her evening feed.
- I checked her blood glucose every two hours during the evening.
- She was hospitalised overnight and her pre-prandial glucose was checked again in the morning. This glucose was 6.7mmol, which is within the normal range (4–10mmol).
- She was sent home later that day. Her owners were advised to continue her normal feeding, exercise and insulin regime.

9. Details of cleaning and maintenance of equipment after use:
to include anaesthetic machine, circuit, endotracheal tube

After surgery I was responsible for carrying out the following:

- The endotracheal tube was rinsed and cleaned with chlorhexidine gluconate. The

tubes were then hung to dry. (Once a week they are sterilised in an appropriate chemical sterilising solution (e.g. Milton), rinsed and hung to dry.)
- The anaesthetic machine is damp dusted every morning and thoroughly disinfected once a week.
- The relevant parts (e.g. corrugated tubing) of the circuits are cleaned and soaked in an appropriate chemical sterilising solution once a week and are daily cleaned of any debris and hung to up to dry.

10. Date of procedure:

15.02.02

Student's Comments and Signature:

This was a very interesting and demanding anaesthetic to monitor because I had to keep a close eye on her blood glucose. I am pleased that Bonnie didn't have any complications during the operation and she recovered rapidly from her anaesthetic and was able to eat.

The evidence in this log sheet and the accompanying record is a true representation of my involvement in the case described, and the work undertaken in compiling this evidence is my own.

Student Veterinary Nurse's Signature:

Assessor's Statement:

The procedures and details associated with the anaesthetic record described on the log sheet and on the attached anaesthetic record have been observed and carried out correctly and competently.

Comments:
Anna demonstrated competence in the monitoring of this anaesthetic. We have discussed the need to express drug doses in mg/ml rather than quantity administered for future case logs to avoid potential confusion.

Assessor's Signature: *Date:*

Assessor's Name: *Assessor's Qualifications:*

LOG SHEET 9C: ANAESTHETIC EMERGENCY BOX

Student Veterinary Nurse's Name:	VN Enrolment No:
A Nonymous	1234

1. Location of the practice anaesthetic emergency box:

The emergency box is located in the prep room, just outside theatre.

2. Contents of the anaesthetic emergency box:

Endotracheal tubes
 – ranging from size 2.5–16mm
Atropine
Doxapram
Heparin saline
Selection of fluids – Hartmann's
 – 0.9% NaCl
 – Mannitol
 – Haemaccel
Tracheostomy tubes

Laryngoscope and blades
Adrenaline 1:1000
Lignocaine
Calcium gluconate
Selection of syringes & needles
Selection of intravenous catheters
Administration sets
Ambu bag
Small surgical kit
Stethoscope

3. Examples of circumstances when each of the drugs or equipment would be used:

Endotracheal tube – to obtain an airway to administer oxygen.
Laryngoscope – to aid placement of ET tube.
Adrenaline – for cardiac arrest, it stimulates the heart and increases blood pressure.
Atropine – to correct bradycardia.
Lignocaine – to treat ventricular arrhythmias.
Doxapram – to stimulate respiration if respiratory failure or apnoea occurs.
Calcium gluconate – used to correct acute hypocalcaemia.
Heparin saline – used to flush intravenous catheters after drug administration or to maintain patency.
Syringes & needles – to administer drugs.
Intravenous catheter – place to obtain immediate intravenous access or administer fluids.
Fluids and administration sets – to restore or maintain circulating blood volume.
Ambu bag – attaches to an ET tube to allow ventilation.
Small surgical kit – for emergency airway access if patient cannot be intubated.
Tracheostomy tubes – to maintain an airway in an emergency.
Stethoscope – to listen for a heart beat or to check the lungs for fluid build-up.

4. Incident when emergency box was used (if applicable):
give brief details of an incident when the emergency box was used and state your role

A cat was recovering from a thyroidectomy. A dressing had been placed around the cat's neck as there had been a lot of postoperative bleeding. Due to the cat not being monitored sufficiently and postoperative swelling the dressing occluded the cat's airway. I found the cat collapsed in its kennel. I immediately called for help recognising that it was an emergency situation. I rushed the cat through to the prep room where I removed the dressing. The veterinary surgeon whose case it was then intubated the cat whilst I assisted by holding its head and neck extended. Once intubated I passed the ambu bag to the vet, who immediately started to ventilate the cat. After a few breaths the cat started to breathe on its own but not sufficiently to take in enough oxygen. The vet asked me to take over ventilation whilst he examined the cat. He checked the cat's heart and femoral pulse which he was happy with. He then checked the cat's pupils to ensure that they constricted and dilated in response to light, which they did. Once the vet had finished his examination he felt that the cat had improved sufficiently for assisted ventilation to stop, so I removed the ambu bag as requested and monitored the cat's breathing. After a further 3–4min the cat was sufficiently recovered to start chewing the ET tube so it was removed. The cat was then placed in a large basket with a vet bed in the prep room so that he could be closely watched. It was my job to take his pulse and respiratory rate every 15min for the first hour of recovery and if anything abnormal happened or I was worried about the cat I was to immediately contact the vet. The cat recovered with no problems and went home the following morning.

5. Date of incident:

28.06.01

Student's Comments and Signature:

From assisting with the above emergency case I learnt the importance of observing your patients closely when they are recovering from operations as things can still go wrong once the ET tube has been removed. It is very important to have an emergency kit so that everything is in one place and is easy to find, so that you can concentrate on the patient and not have to run around wasting time looking for equipment.

The evidence in this log sheet is a true representation of my involvement in the case described, and the work undertaken in compiling the log is my own.

Student Veterinary Nurse's Signature:

Assessor's Statement:

The student has completed the work associated with this log sheet, and has demonstrated practical application and understanding of information provided.

Comments:
Anna's good observation and quick actions helped to prevent the situation deteriorating further. The veterinary surgeon confirmed that Anna was fully aware of her role in this case and competently carried out the procedures requested of her.

Assessor's Signature: *Date:*

Assessor's Name: *Assessor's Qualifications:*

LOG SHEET 10A: MAINTAIN THE SUPPLY OF VETERINARY MATERIALS

Student Veterinary Nurse's Name:	VN Enrolment No:
A Nonymous	1234

1. Name of authorised supplier:

National Veterinary Supplies (NVS)

2. Name of material(s) ordered: *please attach a copy of the order form*

1 x 15kg Hill's canine maintenance
2 x 100ml sodium chloride
4 x 5ml Surolan
1 x 100 5mg Prednisolone tablets
1 x 25 10mg Piriton tablets
1 x 5L Trigene solution

3. Storage of veterinary materials: *please describe how the veterinary materials are stored within your practice and how security of these items is maintained*

Pet food is stored on shelf in the storeroom with a small display in the waiting room. The storeroom is kept locked and a key is kept in the office.

Sodium chloride is stored in a cupboard of injectable solutions alphabetically. Cupboards in the prep room are open all day and locked in the evening.

Surolan is kept in the pharmacy, in the ear treatments cupboard.

Prednisolone and Piriton are stored in the pharmacy. All tablets are kept alphabetically on shelves. Pharmacy is always staffed or locked.

Trigene solution is stored under the sink unit in the prep room, only staff have access.

4. Condition of materials:
please describe how you ensure the condition of veterinary materials is maintained

All material should be stored correctly according to the manufacturer's advice.

Pet food should be stored off the floor in a dry, well-ventilated room.

All drugs should be stored so that the public do not have access to them.

5. Surplus and waste materials:
please describe how surplus and waste materials are disposed of within your practice and state the health and safety requirements relating to such disposal

Clinical waste – includes all waste that consists of animal tissue, blood or other body fluid. It is put into yellow plastic sacks with the words "clinical waste" printed on the outside. It is collected once a week by a company who incinerate it.

Sharps – includes needles, scalpel blades or any sharp instruments. They are discarded immediately after use into special yellow plastic containers that can be sealed once full.

Industrial waste – this is anything that is non-hazardous and is removed by the local council. This waste can go in black sacks.

The principal regulations relating to disposal of waste are:
- Controlled Waste Regulations (1992)
- Control of Pollution Act (1974)
- Environmental Protection Act (1990)

Together the regulations ensure that a practice has correct storage, disposal and destruction of waste.

6. Records of supplies: *please state the method of keeping records relating to the supply of materials and state who has access to these records*

All records are computerised. A copy of each order is printed and kept to cross-reference arrival of goods ordered. The Practice Principal and head nurse who does all the ordering have access to this information. If unpacking an order, you get given a copy of the order to check the order off to ensure that the correct goods have arrived and are in good condition.

Student's Comments and Signature:

From observing and assisting with the orders I feel that I have a greater understanding of the importance of stock control and ensuring that you have enough of all stock.

The evidence in this log sheet is a true representation of my involvement in the case described, and the work undertaken in compiling the log is my own.

Student Veterinary Nurse's Signature:

Assessor's Statement:

Sufficient and reliable evidence has been presented to confirm the student can maintain the supply of veterinary supplies.

Comments:
Anna has assisted in the ordering of supplies and can now deputise in my absence should an order be required. She is also aware of the correct disposal of surplus and waste materials as demonstrated by performance and underpinning knowledge (see Appendix A).

Assessor's Signature: *Date:*

Assessor's Name: *Assessor's Qualifications:*

LOG SHEET 10B: MAINTAIN THE AVAILABILITY OF EQUIPMENT

Student Veterinary Nurse's Name:	VN Enrolment No:
A Nonymous	1234

1. Name of authorised supplier or repairer:

Ritchy Tagg Limited

2. Item(s) of equipment ordered or sent for repair:

Oster A5 clippers

3. Maintenance of equipment:
please describe the general maintenance of the equipment

- I check the clippers every morning and prior to use for the following:
  1. Loose wires
  2. Cracks in the body work
  3. Broken teeth on the blades
  4. Loose screws on blade and clipper body.
- When using the clippers I check that they are cleaned and oiled after each use.
- I also ensure that the blades are disinfected at the end of each day and autoclaved.
- Our clippers are electrically tested on an annual basis by a qualified electrician, as recommended by the Health and Safety Executive.

4. Storage of veterinary supplies: *please describe how the equipment is stored within your practice and how security of such items is maintained*

The clippers are stored in their holders that are screwed to the wall near to a plug socket for ease of use. They are portable and can be moved from room to room within the practice. Specific clippers are designated for outside use for when the veterinary surgeon has to make house calls.

The entire building has a security alarm therefore the clippers are secure from theft from outside personnel.

5. Surplus and waste materials:
please describe how surplus or faulty equipment is disposed of within your practice and state the health and safety requirements relating to such disposal

Any broken blades are disposed of in the sharps bin because they could be sharp but also because they could be contaminated with animal hair and debris from that animal, which is clinical waste.

The two regulations which deal with this are:
- Controlled Waste Regulations (1992)

- The Control of Substances Hazardous to Health (1999)

These state that all sharp instruments should be discarded into special yellow containers that are sealed once full.

6. Records of supplies: *please state the method of keeping records relating to the supply of equipment and state who has access to these records*

All details relating to repair and maintenance of equipment are kept in a book in the practice manager's office. All members of staff have access to this book and record any breakages/failure of equipment or report those breakages/failure in equipment to an appropriate person who should write them in the book.

Any requests for equipment are put in writing to the practice manager in the request book.

Student's Comments and Signature:

I am aware that I am responsible for equipment I use and have to ensure that all the clippers are in full working order at all times. I am happy that I am able to do this, as I have had no complaints from my colleagues.

The evidence in this log sheet is a true representation of my involvement in the case described, and the work undertaken in compiling the log is my own.

Student Veterinary Nurse's Signature:

Assessor's Statement:

Sufficient and reliable evidence has been presented to confirm the student can maintain the availability of veterinary equipment.

Comments:
See case log 8D.

_____

Assessor's Signature: *Date:*

_____

Assessor's Name: *Assessor's Qualifications:*

LOG SHEET 10C: MAINTAIN THE AVAILABILITY
OF VETERINARY EXAMINATION ROOMS

Student Veterinary Nurse's Name:	VN Enrolment No:
A Nonymous	1234

1. Cleaning of examination rooms:

Please provide comments about how the student maintains the cleanliness of examination rooms within the practice.

Anna ensures that the examination table is cleaned between patients and at the end of each surgery she will clean each room. This involves wiping all surfaces down with a dilute disinfectant, restocking items as required (e.g. needles, syringes, cotton wool), sweeping and mopping the floors and checking that all equipment is ready for use.

Once a week Anna cleans the examination rooms thoroughly, all the cupboards and shelves are emptied and cleaned.

Witness' Name: *Date:*

2. Disposal of surplus and waste materials:

Please provide comments about how the student disposes of surplus and waste materials within the veterinary examination rooms.

Anna is very clean and tidy and disposes of any waste immediately. She recognises when it is clinical, sharp or domestic waste and disposes of it appropriately.

Examples of waste materials disposed of:
- Clinical waste – soiled dressings, faeces and empty drug containers.
- Sharps – needles, scalpel blades, any sharp instrument.
- Domestic waste – anything non-hazardous, paper, empty boxes etc.

Witness' Name: *Date:*

3. Equipment and furniture:

Please provide comments about how the student ensures that equipment, materials and furniture are positioned correctly and securely.

Anna ensures that all equipment is always stored in the correct place, therefore reducing the risk of injury. When storing material on shelves she ensures that things are not stacked too high, so that they do not fall off and everything is easily accessible to everyone.

Furniture is not just left lying around, once finished with she places it back in a safe place so that no one comes to any harm.

Examples of areas of work where this occurs:
- In the laboratory when carrying out investigations.
- When working in the prep room with colleagues.
- When putting away orders.

Witness' Name: *Date:*

4. Damage or faults within examination rooms:

Please provide comments about the action the student should take/has taken in the event of identifying damaged or faulty equipment within the examination rooms.

When Anna identifies faulty equipment she reports it to a senior member of staff who deals with the matter. If the equipment cannot be removed from the room she clearly labels it as unsafe and not to use.

Example of any action taken by the student and equipment involved:

Reported a faulty pair of clippers to me as they kept sparking. Anna recognised that the clippers were electrically unsafe and a hazard to use. She removed them from the examination room immediately.

Witness' Name: *Date:*

5. Environmental conditions:

Please provide comments about the environmental conditions the student is able to adjust in order to provide suitable conditions for animals within the examination rooms.

When cats are in examination rooms Anna ensures that all means of escape are shut e.g. windows, doors.

When rabbits, mice, rats etc. are examined Anna has a towel available in case the animal is difficult to handle.

When birds are examined all windows and doors are kept shut to prevent escape.

Witness' Name: *Date:*

6. Security of premises:

Please provide comments about how public and private areas within the practice are identified and how security of private areas is maintained.

Private areas within the practice are identified by signs that have "staff only" clearly written on them.

For extra security such as the kennelling area and radiography room the doors have "no entry" signs on them.

As clients enter the practice there is a sign indicating the waiting area.

Examples of areas restricted to the public:
- Laboratory
- Radiography room
- Kennel area
- Operating theatre

Witness' Name: *Date:*

Student's Comments and Signature:

The evidence in this log sheet is a true representation of my involvement in the case described, and the work undertaken in compiling the log is my own.

Student Veterinary Nurse's Signature:

Assessor's Statement:

Sufficient and reliable evidence has been presented to confirm the student can maintain the availability of examination rooms to provide veterinary services.

Comments:
Anna has demonstrated her competence in the above areas and, on questioning, confirmed that she has good underpinning knowledge relating to element 14.3 of the occupational standards.

Assessor's Signature: *Date:*

Assessor's Name: *Assessor's Qualifications:*

Appendix A: Changes to ATAC approval

Reproduced with permission of RCVS.

Why is there a need to change?

The veterinary nurse training scheme currently has over 1500 approved training and assessment centres (ATACs). Over 1000 of these currently have students in training. Under the current arrangements for ATAC approval, the RCVS is not able to visit practices regularly in order to assure quality, or to provide close support for staff involved in training. Consequently, many practices are working to train nurses in comparative isolation. The RCVS must, as an awarding body for S/NVQs, be able to assure the quality of veterinary nurse training to the Qualifications and Curriculum Authority and Scottish Qualifications Authority (QCA and SQA). It must also be able to satisfy these bodies that practices offering VN training are well supported.

Why is this happening now?

The RCVS has received feedback from practices and its external verifiers that change is necessary. Practices are finding that the mechanisms of assessment and quality assurance (internal verification) are cumbersome and expensive for a single practice to manage. The RCVS recognises that current systems do not allow the awarding body to achieve comprehensive and rigorous quality assurance and that this, in some instances, has led to serious difficulties for student

veterinary nurses. The QCA and SQA audits of veterinary nurse training, conducted in January 2000, confirmed that the current system of ATACs no longer satisfies national requirements and that change is urgently required.

What changes will occur?

In future, there will be several ways in which the RCVS will approve a "centre" for veterinary nurse training. In all cases, the criteria for centre approval will be based upon those stipulated by QCA and SQA. "New" centres may be either a single large veterinary practice or a group of practices acting together in order to provide VN training. There will be several models for these group or consortium-based centres.

What is the aim of the changes?

The changes will enable practices to work together, and in some instances work with course providers

(colleges) in order to provide veterinary nurse training and the resources required to support this. The costs of providing quality assurance of assessment (internal verification) may be shared between a number of practices. Practices new to VN training will have the support of a group of more experienced practices and, in some cases, a course provider. The RCVS will be able to visit each "new" centre (normally twice per year) in order to provide support and monitor the quality of training and assessment.

How will an ATAC train veterinary nurses in the future?

A veterinary practice wishing to train student veterinary nurses may do so in two ways. It may become a veterinary nurse approved centre (VNAC) in its own right or it may join with an approved centre as a training and assessment practice (TP).

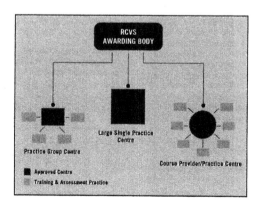

123

What is an approved centre (VNAC)?

An approved centre is either a single veterinary practice or a group (or consortium) of practices working together in order to provide veterinary nurse training and the necessary quality assurance of training and assessment. A consortium-based centre may be a group of independent practices, a commercially linked group of practices or a group of practices working with a veterinary nursing college. In all cases there will be a central point of management and a named principal. However the centre is constituted, it must be able to provide the resources and commitment to veterinary nurse training necessary to satisfy the RCVS criteria for approval. The diagram shows different ways in which an approved centre might be constituted.

What is a training and assessment practice (TP)?

This is a veterinary practice which wishes to train veterinary nurses but does not want, or is not able, to become an approved centre. This may be because the practice is unable to provide all the necessary resources for centre approval or because it wishes to benefit from working in partnership with a larger centre. A TP will recruit and employ student veterinary nurses and manage their training and assessment in much the same way as an ATAC. It will be accountable to the RCVS for quality through its approved centre.

What resources must a training practice have?

A training practice must

have a sufficiently busy and varied caseload for student VNs to be comprehensively trained to the required occupational standards. The standard of the practice premises must also be able to support this training. The RCVS will continue to stipulate the necessary facilities and caseload (which will be similar to those required of an ATAC).

Will a training practice still have to have an assessor?

Yes, your practice must employ a listed veterinary nurse or a veterinary surgeon who is, or is prepared to become, a qualified assessor. This is because S/NVQs must be assessed in the workplace, on the skills being used in everyday clinical practice, rather than in a college. Approved centres must all ensure that their member TPs have assessors, or are able to train them.

In addition, approved centres must ensure that trainee assessors are given adequate support and guidance. This means that many of the difficulties hitherto experienced by veterinary nurses and veterinary surgeons in becoming a qualified assessor will be alleviated.

How does my ATAC or college go about forming an approved centre?

Groups of practices, or a veterinary nurse course provider should contact the Royal College to express an interest in becoming an approved centre (VNAC). The RCVS will forward guidance notes and criteria for centre approval. If the prospective centre is able to meet the required criteria,

an application for approval may be forwarded to the RCVS. Additional guidance will be provided if required by the Veterinary Nursing Department and regional external verifiers. Once an application for approval is received, the RCVS will make arrangements for an approval visit to be made to the prospective centre.

Will the RCVS identify suitable groups of practices for approval as centres?

No, this would be difficult to do because practices will wish to determine for themselves if and how they form groupings in order to provide veterinary nurse training. Even commercially or charitably linked practices will wish to decide whether they will operate as one large (national) centre or as several more locally based centres.

What criteria must an approved centre meet?

The criteria for VNAC approval will be based upon those set by the QCA and the SQA for centre approval. Additionally, the RCVS has specific requirements with regard to the approval and support of member veterinary practices. This will ensure that the overall criteria for S/NVQ centres are met and, in addition, each centre is able to provide and manage suitable clinical training and assessment in veterinary practice.

What happens if my practice wants to be a training practice?

If your practice wishes to train student veterinary nurses and yet is unable, or does not wish, to become

Costs of new VN centre approval

RCVS fees for centre approval	The cost of initial approval of a new centre.	£650
RCVS annual fee	The cost of ongoing quality assurance (external verification).	£400 plus small capitation fee per student
Internal verification	The cost of quality assuring the work of assessors in training practices. Each assessor to be internally verified at least twice per year.	IV time plus travel per visit. Actual cost will depend on size and nature of the centre
Assessment and practical training	This will be provided by training practices. Approved centres must ensure that adequate resources are available and provide support.	Pro-rata salary and training of assessors
Enrolment, tuition and examination fees	These costs will be met by employing TPs as at present.	

RCVS fees must increase to cover the required quality assurance visits and processes. These fees are chargeable only to an approved centre – not to each training practice or to current ATACs.

an approved centre, the practice may join an approved centre as a training and assessment practice (TP). In this case, your practice would apply to an approved centre for membership. The criteria for becoming a TP are simpler than those for ATAC approval (although the clinical and case-load requirements remain similar) and are set for approved centres by the RCVS. The approved centre will arrange to visit your practice prior to accepting you as a member TP. The RCVS will be able to provide you with details of approved centres local to your practice. During the transitional period, when new approved centres are being established, you may find that your practice is approached by a prospective centre seeking member training practices.

What would be the optimum size for an approved centre?

The RCVS does not stipulate a maximum or minimum size for an approved centre. However, a centre must have sufficient resources to be able to meet the QCA and SQA criteria and must also be able to meet the costs of centre approval. This may mean that smaller veterinary practices will have difficulty in providing the necessary resources. These smaller practices may continue to provide good veterinary nurse training through joining with a larger centre. Conversely, a very large centre may find the costs and practicalities of supporting numerous distant member training practices effectively are not viable. Such centres may consider sub-dividing into two or more locally-based smaller centres. It is envisaged that

the majority of veterinary practices will join centres which are able to provide relatively local support (within 30 miles). In remoter areas this distance may extend.

What will be the cost of becoming an approved centre?

The cost of becoming an approved centre for veterinary nurse training will reflect the costs of providing training to VN students and the systems of quality assurance needed to ensure that national standards are met. Costs will vary according to the size of the approved centre and the number of member training practices (for consortium-based centres). The table gives an indication of the nature of approved centre costs; some of which will be shared by member training practices.

Why has the RCVS introduced an annual fee?

This has been introduced to cover the cost of the required external verification visits to every approved centre each year. The current ATAC approval fees do not permit the RCVS to visit on an annual basis as is required. The College will be able to reduce student fees once the new system is in place. This is because external verifiers will be able to sample portfolio assessment during their centre visits. Consequently there should no longer be a need to post these to the RCVS.

What will be the cost to an individual practice training veterinary nurses?

An individual practice which is a member TP of an approved centre will share the costs of quality assurance (the RCVS fees and the cost of internal verification) incurred by their approved centre. The cost of internal verification will vary, depending upon the size of the approved centre but should be in the region of £300 or less per year for a practice with one assessor. Many centres will be able to access TEC or LSC funding to offset these costs. In addition, the training practice will be responsible for the enrolment costs of students and their tuition and examination fees.

If my practice joins with a VN college-based centre, will I be tied to that college for the provision of a VN course?

No, course provision is not tied to centre approval. You may join a college as a member TP and elect to send your student to a different course provider for theoretical instruction. This will enable students and practices to exercise choice as to the most suitable course and mode of delivery.

If I join a consortium-based centre, how will I continue to influence how my veterinary nurses are trained?

The RCVS expects approved centres to have a formal agreement with all member TPs which sets out where responsibilities lie for all aspects of VN training. Within this agreement, clear lines of communication and accountability must be set out. Centres and member TPs are expected to liaise regularly. The RCVS will seek evidence that the training needs and views of practices are sought and acted upon.

Can my practice be a member TP of more than one centre?

Yes, this is possible. However, the practice would incur quality assurance costs from each centre of which it is a member. There should be no reason to join more than one centre.

What happens if I want to change centres?

You would approach your prospective new centre with regard to membership. The new centre will determine, through discussion with you and a visit, whether your practice can meet the RCVS criteria for a TP and is suitable for membership. If so, the practice will be accepted as a member and the RCVS will be informed.

Your "old" centre must also inform the RCVS that you have left.

What happens if a training practice provides poor quality training?

The centre must explore the reasons for poor quality and attempt to achieve a solution through agreement with the TP. The RCVS will require that such action plans are clearly documented and that progress is made towards a solution. Where a breach of quality is very serious, or no immediate solution can be found, the centre must either suspend training at the TP until the problem is resolved or, in the most serious cases, terminate centre membership. In either of these cases the RCVS must be informed.

How will a centre know whether a prospective training practice is a member of another centre or has had membership rejected by another centre?

A centre must always inform the RCVS when a training practice leaves a centre or is not accepted for membership for any reason. The RCVS will keep a record of such moves. Centres may check with the RCVS prior to accepting a new training practice to determine whether membership of any other centre has been refused or terminated, although the actual circumstances will remain confidential.

How will an approved centre ensure that standards of training are maintained?

Each approved centre must satisfy the RCVS that

standards of training and assessment are being maintained and that adequate support is available for nurses in training. A centre will achieve this in several ways:

● The approved centre will ensure that practices joining as TPs have the clinical and personnel resources needed in order to support veterinary nurse training. Centres will visit all prospective TPs in order to ensure that they are able to support training and, in turn, receive the necessary support and guidance from the approved centre.

● An internal verifier (IV) from the centre will visit the practice regularly. The internal verifier will see each assessor in the practice working with a student veterinary nurse at least twice each year in order to ensure that assessment is consistent and meets national standards of good practice. A major function of IV visits will be to provide support and guidance to assessors and to the practice.

● The RCVS will require every approved centre to demonstrate the close support and appropriate management of training practices. The detail of how this is achieved will vary according to the type of centre and the number of member training practices. However, in all cases there must be evidence of regular and effective liaison between the centre and member practices.

● Centres will be expected to provide member training practices with clear criteria for membership and the relationships will be formalised in a written agreement. The RCVS will expect centres to demonstrate how they will be able to identify and deal with a "failing" training practice.

How will the RCVS ensure that standards are being maintained?

The RCVS is required by the regulatory bodies for S and NVQs (SQA and QCA) to ensure that all approved centres are able to meet the awarding body's criteria for centre approval and maintain standards of training and assessment. The College will do this in the following ways:

● An RCVS external verifier (EV) will visit every prospective centre prior to approval being granted to ensure that the required resources and management mechanisms are in place. Where a centre has member training practices, the external verifier will also visit a sample of these practices as part of the centre approval process.

● An external verifier will visit every centre at least twice per year. During these visits the EV will monitor assessment activities (through observing assessment and scrutinising student portfolios) and verify that quality assurance mechanisms are effective. In addition, the overall quality of training and associated student support will be monitored. Where a centre has member training practices, a sample of these will be visited as part of the quality monitoring process.

● The RCVS will maintain a database of all approved centres and their member training practices. Centres will be required to register any new practices joining as member TPs and will also be required to inform RCVS should a member practice leave the centre.

When will these changes take place?

Veterinary nurse course providers and some existing commercially linked veterinary groups will be given the opportunity to become approved centres during early 2001. Once this phase is complete, individual ATACs will be asked to indicate how they wish to proceed. Those practices, or groups, wishing to become centres will apply to the RCVS for approval. Practices wishing to become training practices will seek membership of an approved centre.

The early approval of a core of new VN approved centres will ensure that many practices will have the option to become training practices at an early stage.

The approval of ATACs in 2001 will be for a limited period only (not 5 years). New ATAC approvals will cease by 2002 and all practices training VNs must then either become a new-style VN approved centre or a training practice member of an approved centre. ATAC approval for practices which elect not to become either a training practice or a VN approved centre under the new arrangements will expire once students already in training at the practice have completed the S or NVQ level in progress. Such practices will not be permitted to enrol new students.

Timetable for change

Now onwards	VN course providers (and commercially/charitably linked groups) contact the RCVS for more information.
Early 2001	VN course providers (and other interested groups) sent details of VNAC approval.
Spring 2001	First VNACs approved.
Early Summer 2001	ATACs contacted with details of new VNACs. ATACs indicate to RCVS their intended action.
July 2001 onwards	ATACs join groups or (large ATACS) become new independent centres. RCVS periodically monitors ATAC progress.
July 2002	ATAC approval ends.

My practice has already invested in training an internal verifier; is this wasted?

No, absolutely not. It is a requirement of S and NVQ awards that all assessors must have their work internally verified to ensure consistent and fair standards. If your ATAC becomes a training practice with a new VN approved centre your internal verifier will become part of the centre quality assurance team. If you have a large ATAC and decide to apply for centre approval in your own right, your IV will lead your quality assurance and will be visited at your practice by an RCVS external verifier at least twice per year.

We are about to train an IV, do we still need to do so?

Strictly speaking, yes. However, the changes are being introduced rapidly because the RCVS is aware that many practices have no IV and no immediate plans to make provision for this. If

you plan to join a new VN approved centre as a training practice, the RCVS accepts that you need not take any further action towards internal verifier training at the moment. However, you must actively consider how you will join an approved centre and look for possible partners as soon as details become available in 2001. If your practice is contracting IV services you should continue with these arrangements.

Do we still need to train an assessor?

Yes. Student veterinary nurses must be assessed on their everyday skills in practice. They must have access to a qualified assessor who is able to work alongside them on a regular basis. Training and assessment are closely linked activities and must be co-ordinated by someone who works closely with the student and is aware of their needs and progress. This requirement will not change when the new approval

arrangements commence. Although other S and NVQ training schemes allow for peripatetic assessors to visit students, the RCVS does not believe that such arrangements support quality training.

What do we need to do now?

If you are an ATAC you do not need to do anything just yet, although you will probably be considering which option to take next year. The RCVS will contact you in the early summer of 2001 once the initial network of new VN approved centres is in place.

If you lead an existing group of practices (either charitable or commercial) or are a veterinary nurse course provider you should contact the RCVS as soon as possible if you are interested in becoming a new-style centre. You will be sent further details of the requirements for centre approval and an approval visit will be arranged in the New Year.

Appendix B: Useful names and addresses

British Veterinary Nurse Association (BVNA)
Level 15, Terminus House
Terminus Street
Harlow
Essex CM20 1XA
01279 650567

The College of Animal Welfare
Kings Bush Farm
London Road
Godmanchester
Huntingdon
Cambs PE18 8LJ
01480 831177

Qualifications Curriculum Authority (QCA)
322 Euston Road
London NW1 2BZ
01952 520210

Royal College of Veterinary Surgeons
Belgravia House
62–64 Horseferry Road
London SW1P 2AF
0141 242 2214

Scottish Qualifications Authority (SQA)
Hanover House
24 Douglas Street
Glasgow G2 7N8
020 7222 2001

Appendix C: Further reading

QCA (1996). *Implementing the National Standards for Assessment and Verification.* QCA Publications, Hayes

QCA (1998). *Designing NVQs/SVQs: National Occupational Standards and the Role of the Independent Assessment.* QCA Publications, Hayes

Further copies of the above documents can be obtained by using the QCA Publications Catalogue or by contacting QCA Publications, PO Box 235, Hayes, Middlesex UB3 1HF (telephone 020 8867 3333, fax 020 8867 3233)

Guidance for NVQ/SVQ Awarding Bodies: Disability Discrimination Act 1995. Available from SKILL, National Bureau for Students with Disabilities, 336 Brixton Road, London SW9 7AA

RCVS (1998). *Veterinary Nurse Portfolio Guidance Notes.* RCVS, London

RCVS (1999). *Training Centre Handbook.* RCVS, London

RCVS Veterinary Nursing News. RCVS, London

Centre Point. RCVS, London

TP Times. College of Animal Welfare, Huntingdon, Cambridge

Printed and bound by CPI Group (UK) Ltd, Croydon, CR0 4YY

03/10/2024

01040848-0002